THE
DUKAN
DIET
COOKBOOK

THE
DUKAN
DIET
COOKBOOK

The Essential Companion
to the Dukan Diet

Dr. Pierre Dukan

Crown Archetype

Originally published in France as *Les Recettes Dukan: Mon Regime en 350 Recettes* by Flammarion, Paris, France, in 2007. This translation originally published in slightly different form in paperback in Great Britain as *The Dukan Diet Recipe Book* by Hodder & Stoughton, a Hachette UK Company, London, in 2010.

Library of Congress Cataloging-in-Publication Data
Dukan, Pierre, docteur

  The Dukan diet cookbook : the essential companion to the Dukan diet / Pierre Dukan.
      p. cm.
  "First published in Great Britain in 2010 by Hodder & Stoughton, a Hachette UK Co."—t.p. verso.
  1. Reducing diets—Recipes. 2. High-protein diet—Recipes. I. Title.
  RM222.2.D742 2012
  641.5'63—dc23

                    2012001736

ISBN 978-0-307-98673-3
eISBN 978-0-307-98675-7

PRINTED IN THE UNITED STATES OF AMERICA

Jacket design by Laura Duffy
Jacket photography © Ben Fink
Food stylist: Cyd McDowell
Prop stylist: Sarah Smart

10 9 8 7 6 5 4 3 2 1

FIRST AMERICAN EDITION

CONTENTS

Preface

Taking the Next Step with the Dukan Diet

I wrote the book that you are now holding in France for the French public, and, as perhaps you are aware, the French public is known for two particular cultural features. In addition to being one of the countries most attached to its cuisine and the enjoyment of food, France is also home to some of the world's slimmest women.

I did not conceive this book as a traditional cookbook, focusing solely on flavor and pleasure, but rather as a companion to my Dukan Diet plan—a book full not just of delicious recipes, but of delicious recipes that fit with my golden rules and that use the 100 foods that are allowable on my diet.

When I handed over the manuscript for *The Dukan Diet* to my editor, I was aware that this was the finishing touch to a lifetime's work. The goal of this work had been to provide a method—first for myself, then for my patients, and finally for my future readers—to fight weight problems. The result is my very own method, one that has taken shape over thirty years of daily medical practice and one that has been tried and tested in almost every corner of the world.

When I first started out in the field of nutrition, I, like all my French medical colleagues, was taught that calories counted, and that low-calorie diets, in which every type of food was allowable but in modest quantities, were the way to lose weight. Nowadays, what I know and practice I have learned through direct daily contact with my patients: that low-calorie diets are ineffective for flesh-and-blood human beings, who have constant cravings to eat. It soon became obvious to me that you could not make an overweight person lose weight and stay slim simply by giving them advice to eat less, even if that advice is based on common sense or scientific research.

Dissatisfied with the majority of the diets in vogue, which are only concerned with a dazzling but short-lived victory, and aware of how ineffective low-calorie diets are in reforming overeaters into careful eaters, I developed my own weight-loss diet: the alternating protein diet. Years of medical practice have revealed it to be both the most effective and the most easy-to-follow diet available today, one that delivers the maximum short-, medium-, and long-term results.

The impact of *The Dukan Diet,* the way it has spread, and the affectionate messages I receive from my readers give my life meaning. Whatever my hopes and ambitions may have been when writing my first book, I could never have imagined that it would be so well received by such an incredibly wide and diverse public. The book has been translated and published in countries as distant as Korea, Brazil, and Bulgaria.

How the book spread initially owed very little to marketing and absolutely nothing to advertising. Instead, it sold itself, being passed on from one person to another. From this, I have concluded that the book contained a benefit over and beyond the weight loss results; readers were enjoying the empathy, energy, and experience I bring to my patients as a medical doctor.

As I already mentioned, I have received many letters telling me about results and expressing warmth and gratitude. But I have also received some letters containing criticism or suggestions. Among the latter, some people wanted my weight-loss program to include a section about exercise, and others asked for extra recipes. In the 2011 edition of *The Dukan Diet,* I satisfied this first request with a whole chapter devoted to exercise, one in which exercise is not simply advised, but formally prescribed as medicine. This book, *The Dukan Diet Cookbook,* has been written to satisfy the second request.

For this cookbook, I have been lucky enough to draw upon the inventiveness and contributions of all those people who developed recipes while they were on the diet. For this I am grateful.

And finally I would like to thank you, the reader, for embarking with me on this culinary journey to lasting weight loss.

WHAT IS THE DUKAN DIET?

Proteins and Vegetables— The Foundations of My Diet

For those of you unacquainted with my program or diet, my entire method is based on two main food groups:

- foods rich in animal proteins
- vegetables

These two food categories make up the natural foundation of our human diet. This is because when our species came into being some fifty thousand years ago, our diet consisted of these foods. And to this day, the human body possesses a whole system for digestion and elimination best suited for the foods we ate when we first appeared on earth.

This fact lies at the very heart of my approach. It is not an ideological approach advocating that we return to some backward-looking age, but rather a pragmatic one that recognizes how powerful the inclinations are that are part of our very nature. When our species came into being, man was designed to hunt, to pursue game, and to catch fish. Women concentrated on gathering whatever foods they could find, especially plants. As a result, meat, fish, and vegetables very early on acquired the status of foundation foods, considered the most appropriate foods for humans, both in regard to nutrition and in regard to their emotional power (this being infinitely more useful in weight control). The problem is that for fifty thousand years, these foods have been evolving alongside us.

It is clear that humans are not what they were. No longer hunter-gatherers, people have become sedentary and have learned to grow crops and breed animals. They have built civilizations and brought the environment under their control, so that we can now take from it exactly what we want, including our food, which is now designed far more to be a source of pleasure than a source of nutrition. By doing this, we have created a new diet, poles apart from the one we were designed to eat, and we have become addicted to its voluptuous pleasures. Our new diet appeals to the senses; it is seductive, rich, luscious, and emotionally comforting. But it is a diet that makes us fat.

There are two food groups in our current diet, fats and sugars, that for a long time were found only in foods considered rare and luxurious, but which over the past fifty years have had a dramatic emergence. As a result, our brains and our bodies have come to view these foods with high fat or sugar contents, abundantly available nowadays in supermarkets, as foods of extreme reward. But these foods simply did not exist when our bodies, and in particular our brains, came into being. Nobody ate fats, because the animals that were hunted were lean. Nobody ate sugary foods, because sucrose did not exist.

My intention is not to argue that we return to the caveman's frugal diet, but rather to drive my point home that dieting by going back to eating foods that we originally ate is no hardship. All we need to do is give up our emotional attachment to those high-fat, high-sugar foods and go back to eating the delicious and nutritious foods for which our body was originally made.

Waging the War Against Overeating

I know that most nutritionists advocate that our diet should contain starchy foods, cereals, carbohydrates, and good fats. Thirty years of battling at my patients' side have persuaded me that this sort of diet is difficult to keep up when you are trying to lose weight (though I myself am convinced that slow sugars are useful, but just not during the weight-loss phase). Suggesting to overweight or obese people that they diet by balancing out food groups and limiting portions does not take proper account of their psychology and their issues.

If overweight people were capable of shedding pounds by simply eating a little of everything in a balanced way, they would not have any extra pounds in the first place. Our eating patterns cannot be understood simply through the laws of thermodynamics. This way of explaining excess pounds in terms of energy—people put on weight because they eat too much and exercise too little—is scientifically correct, but it explains nothing about human psychology.

If you have put on weight—to the extent that this extra weight is troubling you—it's likely because, for you, eating fulfills a purpose other than feeding yourself. Although I do not know you personally, I can assure you that whatever it is in your diet that has made you put on weight, it is not what you ate to nourish yourself, but rather the extra things you put in your mouth to give yourself some pleasure. This urge for pleasure can be so strong that it takes you over and drives you to become overweight, even though you end up suffering and feeling guilty because of it.

My daily conversations over the years with patients, listening to them and carefully recording their experiences and stories, have convinced me that if a subconscious demand for pleasure like this exists, an urge that is strong enough to drown out reason and silence feelings of guilt, it is because the person is suffering, temporarily or permanently, from a shortage of other pleasures and other sources of fulfillment. But if you are motivated to do something about your weight, if you have found the energy to wage war against it and to forgo the pleasure you had been getting from the comfort eating that caused your weight problem, you are about to experience an ever greater source of pleasure in your life. That is the pleasure that comes from the promise of brighter, healthier, better days ahead.

During my years of practice, I have seen diets come and go. Analyzing these diets and the reasons behind their incredible success, as well as my own practice, I have observed the strength of my patients' resolve at certain times in their lives. I have also seen how easily they lose heart when the results do not match their efforts. This has convinced me that:

An overweight person who wants to lose weight needs a fast-acting diet that brings immediate results, fast enough to strengthen and maintain his or her motivation.

With this in mind, I have gone for a diet that seems to me today to be both the most appropriate for the particular psychological makeup of overweight people and also the most efficient for weight loss, one that gets fast results, but at the same time adheres to my code of ethics as a doctor. This is to look after my patients' interests over the long term, ensuring permanent and stabilized weight loss.

How a Diet Based on Proteins Evolved

For those of you not acquainted with my diet and who have not yet read *The Dukan Diet,* the work containing my method, I will briefly summarize what is in my program and how it works.

The main focus is on proteins. This is where my journey into the world of nutrition started, and ever since, most of my career as a medical practitioner has been occupied with creating a protein-based diet program.

In 1970, I introduced the first diet in France based solely on this food group. At the time, I had great difficulty getting people to agree to singling out one food group, because it broke completely with the thinking at the time, when low-calorie diets reigned supreme and unchallenged. Nowadays, my protein diet finally has its place among the weapons we use to tackle weight problems. It is the driving force behind any proper diet and to launching the rocket of weight loss.

The prevailing theory, which is extremely conservative and impervious to results and which has been statistically proven time and time again to be wrong, still sides with low-calorie dieting and with eating all foods in tiny quantities. This is a strategy that has produced, still produces, and will forever more continue to produce greater numbers of fat people each year.

Eminent colleagues who hold firm to this position claim that being deprived of certain foods makes us put on weight, that diets that lead to dramatic and sudden weight loss at the outset lead to equally sudden weight gain—often with extra pounds—and unhealthy yo-yoing patterns, especially for first-time dieters. Limiting your diet to certain foods is said to be a surefire way of putting on weight.

I disagree. While such cases do exist, they are far from being the rule. Usually they are due to some frustratingly long and frustratingly low-calorie fad diet, like eating nothing but soup, or the Beverly Hills exotic fruit diet, or a powdered protein diet. This last sort of diet, one restricted to industrially manufactured powders, is doubly damaging, both for our metabolism and for our eating patterns.

The common denominator in all these diets, in which the weight just goes back on again afterward, is the total lack of any stabilization phase. This omission comes both from those advocating the diets, with their token recommendations, such as "be careful," "watch what you eat," "don't overeat," and from people who, still feeling enthusiastic and happy about having lost weight, consider themselves out of all danger. Quite obviously, both sides are mistaken. Only a proper monitoring program can prevent failure and rebounds. And this program must monitor the dieter with precise, concrete, and effective rules that are easy to remember and are part of a ritual. It is this series of graduated rules and responses, acting as a succession of roadblocks to stop you piling back on the pounds, that proves to be enough to control your weight as the weeks and months go by. This is a program that puts you in control and allows you to take action in a comprehensive, concerted, and self-confident way.

The Four-Step Program

The Dukan Diet is a program made up of four successive phases designed to guide overweight people to their desired weight and to keep them there. These four successive phases, which gradually include more foods, have been specially devised to bring about the following results:

- With the first phase, a lightning start and an intense and stimulating weight loss

- With the second phase, a steady, regular weight loss that takes you straight to your desired weight, your own True Weight
- With the third phase, consolidation of this newly achieved but still unstable weight, lasting for a fixed period of time— five days for every pound lost
- With the fourth phase, permanent stabilization, in return for three simple, concrete, guiding, extremely effective but non-negotiable measures to be followed for the rest of your life: protein Thursdays, no more elevators or escalators, and three tablespoons of oat bran *a day*

Each of these phases has a specific effect and a particular mission to accomplish, but all four draw their force and their graduated impact from using pure proteins:

- Pure proteins only during the Attack phase
- Proteins combined with vegetables during the Cruise phase
- Proteins in a more varied diet during Consolidation
- And, finally, one pure protein day a week again in Permanent Stabilization

The Attack phase gets its jump start by using the protein diet in its purest form for two to seven days, depending on the individual.

Alternating pure proteins with proteins and vegetables gives power and rhythm to the Cruise phase, which leads you straight to your desired weight.

The Consolidation phase is the period of transition between hard-line dieting and a return to normal eating.

And finally, the pure protein diet, followed for just one day a week for the rest of your life, guarantees Permanent Stabilization. In exchange for this occasional effort, for the other six days of the week you will be able to eat without guilt or any particular restriction.

How Does the Pure Protein Diet Work?

This Diet Provides Only Proteins

Where Do You Find Pure Proteins? Proteins form the fabric of living matter, both animal and vegetable, so they are found in most known foods. But to develop its unique action and full potential, the protein diet has to be composed of elements as close as possible to pure protein. In practice, other than egg whites, no food is this pure.

Whatever their protein content, vegetables are still too rich in carbohydrates. This includes all cereals, legumes, and starchy foods, and even soybeans—though known for their protein quality, soybeans are too fatty and too rich in carbohydrates.

Some animal proteins are also too high in fat. This is the case with pork; mutton and lamb; some poultry, such as duck and goose; and some cuts of beef and veal.

There are, however, a certain number of foods of animal origin that, without attaining the level of pure protein, come close to it and are the main players in the Dukan Diet.

- Beef, except for ribs, spareribs, and cuts used for braising or stewing
- Lean cuts of veal
- Lean cuts of pork
- Game, such as venison, and some exotic meats, such as ostrich
- Poultry, except for domestic duck and goose
- All fish, including oily fish, which can be included because their fat helps protect the heart and arteries
- All other seafood
- Eggs, even though the small amount of fat in the yolk taints the purity of the egg white
- Fat-free dairy products. Though very rich in protein, they may, nevertheless, contain a small amount of lactose, a natural milk sugar found in milk just as fructose is found in fruit. They can, however, remain in the Dukan Diet's list of allowed foods because they have little lactose but lots of taste.

How Do Proteins Work?

The Purity of Proteins Reduces the Calories They Provide

Every animal species feeds on foods made up of a mixture of the only three known food groups: proteins, carbohydrates, and fats. But for each species, there is a specific ideal proportion for these three food groups. For humans, the proportion is 5-3-2—that is, five parts carbohydrates, three parts fats, and two parts proteins, a composition close to that of mother's milk.

It is when our food intake matches this "golden proportion" that calories are most efficiently assimilated in the small intestine so that it is easy to put on weight.

On the other hand, all you have to do is change this proportion, and the calories are not absorbed as well, and the energy from the foods is reduced. Theoretically, the most radical modification conceivable, which would most drastically reduce the calories absorbed, would be to restrict our food intake to a single food group.

In practice, even though this has been tried out in the United States with carbohydrates (the Beverly Hills Diet allowed only exotic fruits) or fats (the Eskimo Diet), it is hard to eat only sugars or fats, and these have also had serious repercussions for our health. Too much sugar allows diabetes to develop easily, and too much fat poses a major risk to the cardiovascular system. Furthermore, proteins are essential for life, and if the body does not get them, it raids its own muscle for them.

If we are to eat from one single food group, the only possibility is lean proteins: it is a satisfactory solution as far as taste is concerned, it avoids the risk of clogging up the arteries, and by definition it prevents a protein deficiency.

When you manage to introduce a diet limited to protein foods, the body cannot use all the calories contained in the food. It takes the proteins it needs to survive and for the vital maintenance of its organs (muscles, blood cells, skin, hair, nails), and it makes poor and scant use of the other calories provided.

Assimilating Proteins Burns Up a Lot of Calories

To understand the second property of protein, which makes the Dukan Diet so effective, you need to familiarize yourself with the idea of the SDA, or Specific Dynamic Action, of foods. SDA represents the effort or energy that the body has to use to break down food until it is reduced to its basic unit, which is the only form in which it can enter the bloodstream. How much work this involves depends on the food's consistency and molecular structure.

When you eat 100 calories of white sugar, a quick carbohydrate par excellence composed of simple, barely aggregated molecules, the calories are assimilated very quickly. The work to absorb them burns up only 7 calories, so 93 usable calories remain. The SDA for carbohydrates is 7%.

When you eat 100 calories of butter or oil, assimilating them is a bit more laborious: 12 calories are burned up, leaving only 88 for the body. The SDA of lipids is 12%.

Finally, to assimilate 100 calories of pure protein—egg whites, lean fish, or fat-free cottage cheese—the task is enormous. This is because protein is composed of an aggregate of very long chains of molecules, whose basic links, amino acids, are connected to each other by a strong bond that requires a lot more work to be broken down. It takes 30 calories just to assimilate the proteins, leaving only 70 for the body—in other words, the SDA is now 30%. Assimilating proteins makes the body work hard and is responsible for producing heat and raising our body temperature, which is why swimming in cold water after eating a protein-rich meal is inadvisable, as the change in temperature can result in immersion hypothermia.

This characteristic of proteins, while annoying for anyone desperate for a swim, is a blessing for overweight people who are usually so good at absorbing calories. It means they can save calories painlessly and eat more comfortably without any immediate penalty.

At the end of the day, after eating 1,500 calories' worth of proteins, a substantial intake, only 1,050 calories remain after digestion. This is one of the Dukan Diet's key weapons and one of the reasons why it is so effective. But that's not all.

Pure Proteins Reduce Your Appetite

Eating sweet foods or fats, easily digested and assimilated, does create a superficial feeling of satiety, but one that is all too soon swept away by the return of hunger. Recent studies have proved that snacking on sweet or fatty foods does not delay your urge to eat again, or reduce the quantities eaten at the next meal. On the other hand, snacking on proteins does delay your urge for your next meal and does reduce the amount that you then eat. Furthermore, eating only protein foods produces ketonic cells, powerful natural appetite suppressants that are responsible for a lasting feeling of satiety. After two or three days on a pure protein diet, hunger disappears completely, and you can follow the Dukan Diet without the natural threat that weighs down most other diets: hunger.

Pure Proteins Fight Edema and Water Retention

Certain diets or foods are known as being "hydrophilic," that is, they encourage water retention and the swelling this causes. This is the case for mostly vegetable diets, rich in fruits, vegetables, and mineral salts. Protein-rich diets are the exact opposite. They are known as being water-repellent in that they promote elimination through urine and, as such, provide a welcome purge or "drying out" for tissues gorged with water, which is a particular problem during the premenstrual cycle or during perimenopause.

The Attack phase, made up exclusively of proteins that are as pure as possible, best gets rid of water.

This is particularly advantageous for women. When a man gains weight, it is mostly because he overeats and stores his surplus calories in the form of fat. For a woman, how she puts on weight is often more complex and bound up with water retention, which prevents diets from working properly.

At a certain time during the menstrual cycle, in the four or five days before a period starts, or at certain key times in a woman's life—such as puberty, perimenopause, or even in the prime of her sexual life if she has hormonal disorders—women, and especially those who are overweight, begin to retain water and start to feel spongy, swollen, and puffy faced in the morning. They are unable to remove rings from their swollen fingers; their legs feel heavy, and their ankles swell. This weight gain is reversible but it can become chronic.

Even women who diet in order to lose weight and to avoid this swelling are surprised to find that during these periods of hormonal surge, all the little things that worked before no longer have any effect. In all these cases, pure proteins, such as are found in my program's Attack phase, have a decisive and immediate effect. In a few days, sometimes even in a matter of hours, water-soaked tissues begin to dry up, leaving a feeling of well-being and lightness that shows up immediately on the scales and greatly boosts motivation.

Pure Proteins Boost Your Immune System

Before tuberculosis was eradicated through antibiotics, one of the traditional treatments was to overfeed patients by significantly increasing the amount of proteins. At Berck, in northern France, one of the top centers for treating tuberculosis, teenagers were even forced to drink animal blood. Today, sports coaches and trainers advocate a protein-rich diet for athletes who demand a lot from their bodies. Doctors give the same advice to increase resistance to infection, for anemia, or to speed up the healing of wounds.

It is advisable to make use of this advantage, because any weight loss, no matter how small, will weaken the body. I have personally seen that the Dukan Diet's Attack phase is the most stimulating phase. Some patients have even told me that it had a euphoric effect, both mentally and physically, and that this happened from the end of the second day.

Pure Proteins Enable You to Lose Weight Without Losing Muscle or Skin Tone

There is nothing surprising in this observation when you realize that the skin's elastic tissue, as well as muscle, is made up essentially of proteins. A diet lacking in proteins forces the body to use its own muscles and the skin's proteins, so that the skin loses its elasticity. Combined, these effects cause aging of the skin, hair, and even general appearance, which friends and family soon notice, and which can be enough to make you stop the diet early. Conversely, a protein-rich diet and, even more so, a diet made up exclusively of proteins like the Dukan Diet's Attack phase, has no reason to attack the body's reserves because the body is being given substantial protein supplies. Under these conditions, the weight loss is rapid, muscle firmness is maintained, and the skin glows, allowing you to lose weight without looking older.

This particular feature of the Dukan Diet might seem of secondary significance to young women with firm muscles and wrinkle-free skin, but it is very important for those women approaching their fifties, and therefore menopause, or for those who have less muscle structure or fine and delicate skin. This is especially important because there are too many women nowadays who manage their figures guided solely by their scales. Weight cannot and should not be the sole issue. Radiant skin, healthy-looking hair, tissue strength, and general body tone are criteria that contribute just as much to a woman's appearance.

Conclusion

The pure protein diet, the initial and principal driving force behind the four integrated diets that make up my program, is not like other diets. It is the only one to use just a single food group and one well-established category of foods with the highest protein content.

During this diet and throughout the whole program, any mention of calories and of calorie counting is to be avoided. Whether a few or many calories are eaten has little effect on the results. What counts is keeping within this food category. So the actual secret of the program's first two weight-loss phases is to eat a lot, even to eat in anticipation, before the hunger pangs take over. Hunger that turns into uncontrollable cravings that can no longer be appeased by the proteins you are allowed to eat leads the careless dieter toward pure comfort foods with little nutritional value—sugary, creamy, rich, and destabilizing foods that nevertheless have a strong emotional power.

By following this diet, you have replaced a calories system with a categories system. There is absolutely no need for you to count calories;

all you need do is stay within the categories. But if you stray from the list of permitted foods, you are no longer allowed to eat any quantity you like, and you will have to start counting how many calories you eat.

So this is a diet you cannot follow in half measures. It relies on the great all-or-nothing law, which explains not only its metabolic effectiveness, but also its amazing impact on the psychology of an overweight person.

THE 100 NATURAL FOODS FOR THE ATTACK AND CRUISE PHASES

Eat as Much as You Like

My method consists of four phases, and I have used this structure to organize the recipes. The first two phases, the Attack and the Cruise phases, are responsible for actual weight loss. The next two phases, the Consolidation and the Stabilization phases, maintain the weight loss you have achieved.

Recipes have the most vital role to play during the first two phases: to offer pleasure, flavor, and variety, and to satisfy hunger. Afterward, so much diversity is possible that no single book could contain all the recipes. However, in this book you will find two types of recipes, all of which can be eaten during the Attack and the Cruise phases:

- Recipes that we call "pure protein recipes" because they use only foods with a high protein content. These recipes can be used for all phases of the diet, but are the only recipes to be used in the Attack phase.

- Recipes that combine proteins and vegetables. These recipes can be used in the Cruise phase.

These recipes have been devised based on the 100 foods that make up my diet, and there is absolutely no restriction on how much you can eat, when, and in what combination. You are granted this total freedom on condition that you introduce no other food during the program's first two phases, which will take you to the weight you want.

In the first two phases of my program, you can eat as much as you like of the following 100 foods:

Protein Foods (Attack) Phase

Lean Meats and Organ Meats

By lean meat, I mean beef, veal, lean pork, and game.

- Beef: All roasts or grilled beef is allowed—namely, steaks, tenderloin, sirloin, and roast beef; you must carefully avoid all types of ribs, as they are too fatty.
- Veal: Recommended are veal cutlets and roast veal; veal chops are allowed as long as you trim all the fat.
- Pork: Lean cuts of pork, such as tenderloin, loin roast, or well-trimmed center-cut chops are permitted.
- Game: Buffalo and venison are permitted.
- Lamb: Lamb is not allowed in the Attack phase.
- Liver (beef, veal, or poultry) and tongue: Liver is rich in vitamins, which are very useful during a diet. Unfortunately, liver is also high in cholesterol, so it should be avoided if you have any cardiovascular problems.

Fish

There is no restriction or limitation with this family of foods. All fish are allowed, lean or fat, white or oily, fresh, frozen, dried, smoked, or canned (but not in oil or sauce containing fat).

- All fatty fish and oily fish are allowed, such as sardines, mackerel, bluefish, tuna, and salmon.
- All white and lean fish are also allowed, such as sole, halibut, cod, sea bass, mahi-mahi, tilapia, orange roughy, catfish, perch, skate, trout, flounder, and monkfish, as well as many other lesser-known varieties.
- Smoked fish is permitted, too; smoked salmon, although greasy looking, is less fatty than a 90 percent fat-free steak. The same goes for smoked trout, tuna, eel, and haddock.
- Canned fish, very handy for quick meals or picnics, is allowed if it is packed in brine or in water, like tuna, salmon, and mackerel; sardines packed in tomato sauce are also allowed.
- Finally, you are allowed to have surimi. Originally from Japan, these crab sticks are made with very lean white-fleshed fish and are flavored with crab sauce and a little sugar. Many of my readers have an unfavorable opinion of them. It is true that this is a processed food, but having researched into how it is produced, I have seen that it is of high nutritional quality, prepared from small white fish on factory ships on the open sea. Others have pointed out to me that the labels mention carbohydrates. This is true, but that does not rule them out as the carbohydrate is in the form of starch, which can be tolerated because of surimi's other qualities. The fat content is in fact very low.

Shellfish

Here I include crustaceans and all shellfish.

- Shrimp, crayfish, crab, lobster, scallops, oysters, clams, and mussels, as well as squid and octopus.

Poultry

- All poultry is allowed except birds with flat beaks, such as farm-reared goose and duck, provided you do not eat the skin. You can leave the skin on when cooking and remove it on your plate at the last moment so that the meat does not dry out.
- Chicken is the most popular poultry product and the most practical one for the pure protein Attack phase. Everything is allowed except the outside part of the wings, which is too fatty and cannot be separated from the skin. However, you should be aware that different parts of the chicken have differing amounts of fat. The leanest part is the white breast meat, followed by the thigh, then the wing. Finally, the chicken should be as young as possible.
- Turkey in all forms is allowed, as are Cornish hens and quail. If you have access to game birds such as pheasant and wild duck, which is lean, they are also permitted.

Eggs

Hen's eggs or quail's eggs can be eaten hard-boiled, soft-boiled, poached, or in an omelet, but always without any butter or oil. Unless you are sure of the source of your eggs, they should be cooked through; undercooked eggs carry the risk of salmonella. If you have access to pasteurized eggs, this will not be an issue.

To make your eggs more sophisticated and less monotonous, you can add shrimp or even some shredded crab. Try omelets with chopped onion or a few asparagus tips just for the flavor, ham, and spices. In a diet where quantities are not restricted, eggs can be problematic because they are high in the cholesterol they contain in their yolks. Excessive consumption should be avoided by anyone with a high cholesterol level in their blood; in such cases, no more than three or four egg yolks should be eaten per week. But the egg white, a pure protein par excellence, can be eaten without restriction. You can make omelets using just one yolk for every two whites. Some people are allergic to eggs; of course, they should avoid them.

So, if you are not allergic to eggs and do not have a high cholesterol count, and if you cook them without oil or butter, you may eat two eggs every day without running any risk during this brief Dukan Diet Attack period.

Fat-Free Dairy Products (Fat-Free Yogurt, Fat-Free Sour Cream, Fat-Free Cream Cheese, Fat-Free Cottage Cheese)

These foods were developed to make losing weight easier. Just as the transformation of milk into cheese is responsible for the elimination of lactose, the only sugar found in milk, these fat-free dairy products contain practically nothing but protein, which is why they are so useful when we are looking for pure proteins during the Attack phase.

For some years now, milk producers have sold a new generation of yogurts sweetened with aspartame or Splenda or enriched with fruit pulp. While artificial sweeteners and other flavorings have no calorie content, the added fruit introduces unwanted carbohydrates. This drawback is compensated for by the fact that these gratifying treats give you the opportunity to enjoy a sweet and so can help you follow the overall diet program. So that the instruction is clear, there are three sorts of fat-free yogurt: natural yogurt; flavored yogurts, such as coconut, vanilla, lemon; and fruit yogurts with little bits of fruit or a fruit purée base.

- Natural and flavored fat-free yogurts are both allowed without any restriction.
- Fat-free fruit yogurts are allowed, but no more than 8 ounces per day. However, if you want a lightning-fast start to your Attack phase diet, you are better off avoiding them altogether, and even more so if you are going through a period when your weight is plateauing.

Vegetable Protein

In the last decade, I have noticed a reduction in the appetite for meat, especially among women. Vegetable proteins come from soy and wheat (gluten); most of these vegetable proteins are from Asia, in particular Japan.

Here I will discuss seven vegetable-protein foods that are very high in protein and low in fat. However, only the first two—tofu and seitan—have the relationship between proteins, fats, and carbohydrates that allows them to be used in unlimited quantities, like the foods in the six previous categories. The last five—tempeh, soy steaks and vegetable burgers, textured soy proteins, soy milk, and soy yogurt—are foods that I would, however, reserve only for vegetarian readers who do not consume meat or fish. For nonvegetarians, these five foods are to be used as Tolerated Foods (see page 30), the use of which is subject to weight and frequency conditions.

Tofu Tofu comes in several forms (the most common are silken and firm or extra-firm) and is widely available in supermarkets as well as natural and health food stores.

Silken tofu has the consistency of flan or yogurt. It can be found either with the refrigerated vegetables or in the dairy case. It is useful in making dessert and pastry recipes and for quiches based on oat bran galettes. It is also an interesting alternative in the preparation of sauces to replace mayonnaise, yogurt, or sour cream. Its consistency means that it can be whipped to act as a cream substitute.

Firm (or extra-firm) tofu has the consistency of semisoft cheese. It can be used in various forms: crumbled, grated, in small chunks, or as a purée for all kinds of main dishes, starters, and desserts. It is naturally tasteless but soaks up all the flavors of the foods surrounding it. It combines very well with chives, soy sauce, and mild spices. Use it in chunks in mixed salads or in vegetable tarts made with oat bran.

Tofu benefits enormously from being marinated in the sauce of your choice for a few hours before cooking. To allow it to better soak up the flavor of the marinade, be sure to press it between two plates, using a weight to remove excess water.

Firm tofu is stored like mozzarella, refrigerated in water, which should be changed every two days, and can be stored for not more than ten days.

Tofu holds a favored position in the Dukan Diet. You can now find herbed tofu, curried tofu, and smoked tofu. You can also find tofu dumplings, vegetarian sausages, stir-fries, and raviolis made with tofu, all of very high quality and great flavor.

A word of warning! Not all these dishes and presentations have been cooked in accordance with our dieting requirements, and you should look closely at their labeling in order to avoid those with a fat content of over 8 percent.

Seitan Seitan, or "vegetable meat," is made with wheat proteins rather than soy proteins. Its resistant texture is reminiscent of meat, which allows it to be used in stews, prepared on skewers, or braised.

Seitan can be found ready to use, natural or flavored, in natural and health food stores, Asian markets, and some well-stocked supermarkets. While used primarily by vegetarians and vegans as a source of protein, I think that it is high time for it to be introduced to a wider audience, especially to people who are trying to lose weight.

On a nutritional level, seitan is a food extremely rich in protein (25 percent) and low in calories (110 calories per 100 grams); it contains very few carbohydrates, almost no fat and no cholesterol.

Use seitan by the date on the package; it can also be frozen for longer storage.

If you are cooking seitan, to prevent it from becoming hard, cook it covered on low heat, rather than quick-frying it. It is better to pan-fry it gently, so that it becomes more tender. To maintain its best consistency and flavor, avoid using slices that are too thick. Think about marinating it in a mix of soy sauce, herbs, spices, and low-sodium chicken broth before adding it to the pan. You will find a number of delicious recipes for seitan on our website, www.dukandiet.com.

Tempeh Of Indonesian origin, tempeh is made by fermenting soybeans. Tempeh has a firm texture and a natural nutty mushroom taste. It is rich in protein, with a low fat content and no cholesterol. It is a choice food for vegetarians.

A word of warning! Tempeh's carbohydrate content limits its place in my diet, where it can only be used as a Tolerated Food.

Soy Steaks and Vegetable Burgers Soy steaks and vegetable burgers are useful mostly to vegetarians who do not eat meat. It is essential to read the labels, as the fat content can vary from single to double digits. A very large variety of these products is sold by the large food retailers, as well as pre-prepared cooked meals. The disadvantage of this wide choice of brands and flavors is the mix of very different ingredients. Some burgers are soy based; others are based on cereals or on vegetables. This variety has a big impact on the nutritional composition. Also, it is important to consult the label to check the carbohydrate content, which is the limiting factor in my diet. I have selected two brands from among the most widely used products, Boca and MorningStar.

- From Boca, choose Boca Grilled Vegetable, Boca All American Flame Grilled, Boca Original Vegan, or Boca Cheeseburger.
- From MorningStar, choose MorningStar Farms Classic Burger made with Organic Soy or MorningStar Farms Grillers.

Textured Soy Proteins, or TSP Textured soy proteins are prepared using de-oiled soy flour that is mixed with water and heated under pressure. The mix is then dried and broken up into granules or larger pieces.

Textured soy proteins have numerous advantages. They contain twice as much protein as beef. They are low in calories and do not contain cholesterol. They can be easily stored and can be kept for a very long time. Finally, they are very good value and easy to cook. Their texture is similar to meat and they are designed to be hydrated and prepared in the same way as meat. In their raw state, they have a crunchy consistency and a hint of peanut flavor, which makes them very appealing as a snack.

A word of warning! In my diet, as is the case for tempeh, their carbohydrate content means that they can only be used as a Tolerated Food.

Soy Milk Soy milk is a nondairy drink high in vegetable proteins and low in calories, carbohydrates, calcium, and vitamin D. It does not contain cholesterol.

Soy milk can be used as a milk substitute for individuals who do not drink cow's milk: vegetarians and people who are lactose-intolerant, do not like the taste of cow's milk, or have a tendency toward high cholesterol.

Soy milk can be drunk plain or flavored and can be used to make all kinds of sauces usually based on milk, such as béchamel sauce.

A word of warning! In the context of my diet, you are limited to two glasses of unsweetened soy milk per day, to replace fat-free cow's milk.

Soy Yogurt Soy yogurt is made from soy milk and has the same characteristics. It offers an alternative to all those who are allergic to lactose or who have difficulty digesting dairy products, or who are pure vegans.

With regard to its nutritional and calorific value, it is very similar to low-fat milk yogurt, with an average fat content of 2 percent depending on the brand, but cholesterol-free.

You are permitted two 6-ounce natural soy yogurts (no sugar) per day.

Vegetables (Cruise Phase)

In the Cruise phase, as well as protein-rich foods, you are allowed all cooked or raw vegetables without restriction regarding quantity, time of day, or combination.

You can eat tomatoes, cucumbers, radishes, spinach, asparagus, leeks, green beans, cabbage, mushrooms, celery, fennel, eggplant, zucchini, summer squash, peppers, all types of lettuce, and even carrots and beets, provided you do not have them at every meal.

Vegetables considered to be starchy foods are, however, forbidden: potatoes, corn, fresh or dried peas, beans, and lentils. Avocado is also forbidden; it is not a vegetable, but a fruit, and a very fatty fruit in the bargain. Rice, quinoa, barley, wheat berries, millet, and other grains are not allowed.

How Should These Vegetables Be Prepared—Raw or Cooked? For everyone who can digest raw vegetables, it is always preferable to eat vegetables when they are fresh and uncooked so that you do not lose any of the vitamins they contain.

Oat Bran

For years, the first two actual weight-loss phases in my program did not contain any starchy foods, cereals, or flour-based foods. The program worked fine without them, but many of the men and women who followed it eventually ended up longing for carbohydrates.

I discovered oat bran while attending a cardiology conference in America, where there was a presentation on how it reduces cholesterol and diabetes. I brought some home, and one morning, having run out of flour, I created a special pancake, which I now call the Dukan Oat Bran Galette, for my daughter, Maya. It is made of oat bran, an egg white, and fat-free plain Greek-style yogurt, sweetened with a zero-calorie sweetener suited for cooking or baking. As she loved it and felt completely full, this spurred me on to suggest to my patients that they try the galette. Their enthusiasm for it persuaded me to include it in my method and my books. This is how oat bran gradually became a fundamental part of my method. It is the only carbohydrate allowed among the proteins and even within the sanctuary of the Attack phase. Why?

First, from a clinical perspective, I very quickly noticed an improvement in results: my patients followed the diet better over the long term; they felt less hungry and full sooner; and all in all, they were much less frustrated.

I tried to understand how oat bran works and looked at the studies available on it. Oat bran is the fibrous husk that surrounds and protects the oat grain. The grain, used to make rolled oats, is rich in simple sugars. Oat bran is the grain's jacket. It has few simple sugars but is very rich in proteins and particularly in soluble fibers. These fibers have two physical properties that give oat bran its therapeutic role.

Oat bran can absorb, on average, up to twenty-five times its volume in water. This means that as soon as it reaches the stomach, it swells up and takes up enough space to make you very quickly feel full. It is also extremely high in soluble fiber and can reduce the absorption of dietary fat.

Because oat bran makes you feel full and pushes food through your system more quickly, it is a precious ally in my battle against the weight problem epidemic.

I have done my own research on oat bran and have found that the way the bran is produced greatly determines how effective it is. Two manufacturing parameters, milling and sifting, turned out to be crucial. Milling involves grinding the bran and determines the size of its particles; sifting involves separating the bran from the oat flour.

If the milling is too fine, the bran loses almost all its effectiveness. Likewise, if the bran is too coarse, its useful surface viscosity is lost. If the bran is not thoroughly sifted, it is not sufficiently pure and contains too much flour.

Milling should ideally produce particles with a medium+ size (technically called M2bis). As for sifting, it is after it has been sifted for a sixth time, B6, that oat bran has negligible fast carbohydrate content. These two indexes together make up the overall M2bis-B6 index.

I am currently working with international manufacturers and distributors, sharing these results with them to try to get them to adopt the milling-sifting index, which makes production a little more expensive but produces more nutritional bran. In the meantime, the recommended type of oat bran, Dukan Diet Organic Oat Bran, can be found on our website, www.shopdukandiet.com.

During the Attack phase, I prescribe 1½ tablespoons of oat bran per day. I recommend eating it as prepared in the Dukan Oat Bran Galette.

Dukan Oat Bran Galette

This light and easy pancake is a tasty way to eat your oat bran.

MAKES 1 GALETTE

Preparation time: 10 minutes

Cooking time: 10 minutes

2 tablespoons oat bran, such as Dukan Diet Organic Oat Bran

2 tablespoons fat-free plain Greek-style yogurt

1 teaspoon zero-calorie sweetener suited for cooking and baking, such as Splenda, for a sweet pancake

or

Freshly ground black pepper, herbs, and/or chopped garlic for a savory pancake

1 egg white

1. In a medium bowl, combine the oat bran and yogurt with the sweetener for a sweet pancake, *or* with the pepper, herbs, and/or garlic for a savory pancake.
2. In a separate bowl, beat the egg white until foamy.

3. Fold the beaten egg white into the oat bran mixture until blended.

4. Heat a small nonstick frying pan over medium heat. Pour the mixture into the hot pan and cook until the underside is golden and the upper side starts to dry, about 5 minutes.

5. Using a spatula, flip the galette and continue cooking the other side until browned, about 5 more minutes.

6. Remove the galette to a plate and allow to cool briefly before serving.

Most of my patients eat their galette for breakfast, so that they avoid feeling famished midmorning. Others eat the galette for lunch with a nice slice of smoked salmon or some thinly sliced ham or turkey breast. Other patients have the galette in late afternoon, at the "danger hour," when cravings can overtake them, or even after supper, when they want to rummage around in the cupboard to find a final treat before bedtime. If you would like some more oat bran–based ideas, see the www.all aboutoatbranusa.com website for a whole range of recipes for crêpes, muffins, cakes, pizza bases, and oat bran bread.

If you are going through a difficult period when irrepressible cravings are overwhelming, for a day or two (and I really do mean for a day or two), you can eat more oat bran and up to three galettes per day.

Discover Dukan Diet Organic Oat Bran

Tolerated Foods

Tolerated foods are specific foods permitted in calibrated portions when weight loss is steady and satisfactory. They should be avoided during periods of weight-loss stagnation.

In the Cruise phase, two tolerated foods are permitted per day; three tolerated foods are permitted in the Consolidation phase, except on Protein Thursdays.

Fat-free yogurt with fruit, 1 serving

Plain fat-free DanActive, 1 serving

Reduced or fat-free heavy cream, 1 tablespoon

Plain soy yogurt, 1 serving

Cheese, at least 93% fat-free, 1 ounce

Fat-free sour cream, 1 teaspoon

Soy milk, 1 cup

Soy flour or cornstarch, 1 tablespoon

Goji berries, per day: 1 tablespoon during the Attack phase and on Pure Protein days during the Cruise phase; 2 tablespoons on Protein+Vegetable days of the Cruise phase; 3 tablespoons during the Consolidation phase

Flax seeds, 1 teaspoon

Chia seeds, 1 teaspoon

Chicken or turkey sausage, at least 90% fat-free, 3½ ounces

Cooking wine, uncovered when cooking so it evaporates, 3 tablespoons

Worcestershire sauce, 1 teaspoon

Nonfat sugar-free cocoa, at least 90% fat-free such as Dukan Diet Organic Cocoa Powder, 1 teaspoon

The Problem with Dressings

Dressings may appear harmless, but they are a major problem for weight-loss diets. Indeed, many people base their diet on salads and crudités, which are low in calories and rich in fiber and vitamins. This is perfectly true, but do not forget that it is the dressing that upsets the balance of these good qualities. Let's take a simple example: in an ordinary salad bowl containing 2 heads of lettuce and 2 tablespoons of oil, the salad accounts for 20 calories and the oil for 200 calories, which is why so many diets based on mixed salads fail.

We also need to clear up the ambiguity concerning olive oil. Even though this symbol of the Mediterranean lifestyle is recognized as protecting us against cardiovascular disease, it is no less rich in calories than any other oil on the market.

For these reasons, during the first two actual weight-loss phases, the

Attack and Cruise phases, it is crucial that you avoid preparing green vegetables, cooked or raw, with a sauce or dressing that contains more than 1 teaspoon of vegetable oil.

Vinaigrette
Here is an easy, flavorful vinaigrette that uses a tiny amount of oil.

In a clean, empty jar, combine 1 tablespoon mustard (Dijon or, even better, French whole-grain mustard), 5 tablespoons balsamic vinegar, 1 teaspoon vegetable oil, and salt and freshly ground black pepper to taste. If you like garlic, add a large clove to marinate in the bottom of the jar, together with 7 or 8 fresh basil leaves. Cover the jar and shake vigorously to mix the dressing before serving. If using the garlic, set the jar aside for 30 minutes to infuse the dressing with the garlic and remove the garlic before serving.

If you do not like balsamic vinegar, that is a pity, as it is more appealing to the senses, but you can select another one. Just use a little less: 4 tablespoons for wine, sherry, or raspberry vinegar; 3 tablespoons for champagne vinegar.

Vinegar is a condiment that can play a major role in any diet. An interesting paradox has recently been discovered: that humans can distinguish four universal flavors—sweet, salty, bitter, and sour—yet vinegar is the only substance in the human food list to provide that precious and rare sour taste.

Moreover, recent studies have also demonstrated the impact that oral sensation—the quantity and the variety of flavors—has on producing the feeling of satisfaction and fullness. For example, we know today that the taste of certain spices—such as cloves, ginger, turmeric, star anise, and cardamom—work on the hypothalamus, the area in our brain that measures these sensations until the feeling of satiety is triggered. So it is very important to use as wide a range of spices and as much as possible, preferably at the start of a meal, and, if you are not already a great fan, to try to get used to them.

Yogurt Dressing

It is also easy to make a savory sauce with fat-free plain Greek-style yogurt. Add 1 tablespoon of mustard (Dijon, if possible) to 6 to 8 ounces of yogurt and beat the mixture together until it has the consistency of mayonnaise. Add a dash of vinegar and some salt, freshly ground black pepper, and herbs.

The Importance of Drinking Water

Opinions and rumors circulate about how much water you should drink, but almost always there is some kind of "authority" telling you today the exact opposite of what you heard yesterday. However, this water issue is not simply a marketing concept for diets; it is a question of great importance.

To simplify things, it may seem essential to burn calories so that our fat reserves melt away; but this combustion, as necessary as it is, is not enough. Losing weight is as much about eliminating waste as it is about burning fat.

Would you do a load of laundry or wash the dishes without rinsing them? It is the same with losing weight. A diet that does not involve drinking a sufficient quantity of water is a bad diet. Not only is it ineffective, it leads to the accumulation of harmful waste.

Water Purifies the Body and Improves the Diet's Results

Simple observation shows us that the more water you drink, the more you urinate and the greater the opportunity for the kidneys to eliminate waste derived from the food burned. Water is, therefore, the best natural diuretic. It is surprising how few people drink enough water.

The many demands in our busy day conspire to delay, then finally eliminate, our natural feeling of thirst, which no longer plays its part in warning us about tissue dehydration. Because their bladders are smaller and more sensitive than men's, many women do not drink to avoid having to go to the bathroom constantly, or because it is awkward at work or on public transport, or because they do not like public restrooms.

However, what you may get away with under ordinary circumstances has to change when following a weight-loss diet.

Trying to lose weight without drinking is not only toxic for the body; it can reduce and even completely block the weight loss so that all your work is for nothing. Why?

Because the human engine that burns its fat while dieting functions like any combustion engine. Burned fuel (proteins) gives off heat and waste. If these waste products are not regularly eliminated by the kidneys, they will accumulate and, sooner or later, interrupt combustion and prevent any weight loss, even if you are following the diet scrupulously.

It is the same for a car engine with a clogged exhaust pipe, or a fire in a fireplace full of ashes. Both end up choking and dying from the buildup of waste. Sooner or later, bad nutrition and the accumulated effects of bad health care and extreme or unbalanced diets will make the overweight person's kidneys become lazy. More than anyone else, overweight people need large quantities of water to get their kidneys working efficiently again.

At the outset, drinking a lot of water may seem tedious and unpleasant, especially in wintertime. But if you keep it up, the habit will grow on you. Then, encouraged by the pleasant feeling of cleaning out your insides and, even better, of losing weight, drinking water often ends up once again becoming something you need to do.

When Should You Drink Water?

People still cling to old wives' tales that would have you believe that it is best not to drink at mealtimes to avoid food trapping the water. Not only does this idea have no physiological basis, in many cases it makes things worse. Not drinking when you eat, at a time when you naturally get thirsty and when drinking is so easy and enjoyable, may contribute to suppressing your thirst. Then, when you are busy later on with your daily activities, you may forget to drink water for the rest of the day. During the Dukan Diet, and especially during the alternating proteins (Cruise) phase, except in cases of exceptional water retention caused by hormonal or kidney problems, it is absolutely essential to drink 1½ quarts of water a day. If possible, drink mineral water or take water in any other liquid form, such as tea, herbal tea, or coffee.

Have a cup of tea at breakfast, a large glass of water midmorning, 2 more glasses and a coffee at lunch, 1 glass during the afternoon and 2 glasses with dinner, and you have easily downed 2 quarts. Many patients have told me that in order to drink when they were not thirsty, they got into the habit of drinking directly from the bottle, and this worked better for them.

Which Water Should You Drink?

- *Mineral water.* The most suitable waters for the pure protein Attack phase are mineral waters low in sodium, which are slightly diuretic and laxative. Among the best-known mineral waters are Evian, Poland Spring, Fiji Water, Voss, Saratoga Spring, and Perrier, the famous sparkling variety. You should avoid San Pellegrino, which is good but contains too much sodium to be drunk in large quantities.
- *Tap water.* If you drink tap water, then continue to do so. It is far more important to drink enough water to get your kidneys working again than it is to worry about what is in the water you are drinking.
- *Tea.* The same holds true for all the various sorts of teas, green teas, and herbal teas, especially in colder weather.
- *Diet soda.* In the case of diet sodas, I consider them all to be great allies in the fight against weight problems (or excess weight) as long as they have no more than 1 calorie per glass. As far as I am concerned not only do I allow them, I recommend them and for several reasons.

  First of all, diet sodas are often the best way to make sure you drink the 1½ quarts of liquid already mentioned. In addition, they have virtually no calories or sugar. Finally, and above all, a carbonated beverage like Diet Coke or Coca-Cola Zero, the market-leading brand, provides a clever mix of intense flavors, just like traditional Coke, which can reduce the craving for sugar if used repeatedly by those who like snacking on sweet things.

Many of my patients have confirmed that diet sodas were fun and comforting when used as a part of their diet and actually helped them. The sole exception regarding diet sodas is in the case of a dieting child or teenager. It has been proved that substituting "fake" sugar does not work and barely reduces their craving for sugar. Furthermore, unlimited use of sweet-tasting carbonated drinks might form a habit of drinking without thirst and just for pleasure.

Water Is Naturally Filling

As you know, we often associate the sensation of an empty stomach with being hungry, which is not entirely wrong. Water drunk during a meal and mixed with food increases the total volume of the food mass and stretches the stomach, creating a feeling of fullness, the first sign of satisfaction and satiety—yet another reason for drinking at mealtimes. However, experience proves that keeping the mouth busy works just as well in between meals, for example during the danger zone in your day, between 5 p.m. and 8 p.m. A big glass of any liquid will often be enough to calm your hunger pangs.

Nowadays, the world's richest populations are confronting a new type of hunger: a self-imposed denial while surrounded by an infinite variety of foods they dare not touch because of the risk to their health or because they have weight problems.

It is surprising to see that at a time when individuals, institutions, and pharmaceutical laboratories dream of discovering the perfect and most effective appetite suppressant, there are so many people for whom this is an issue who still do not know about or, even worse, refuse to use a method as simple, pure, and inexpensive as drinking water to tame their appetite.

The Diet Has to Be Low in Salt

Kicking the Salt Habit

Salt is an element vital to life and present to varying degrees in every food, so adding salt at the table is always superfluous. Salt is just a condiment that improves the flavor of food, sharpens the appetite, and is all too often used purely out of habit.

A low-sodium diet is never dangerous. You could and even should live your whole life on a low-sodium diet. People with heart and kidney problems or high blood pressure live permanently on low-sodium diets without suffering harmful effects. However, people with natural low blood pressure and those who are used to using salt on their food should exercise caution.

A diet too low in salt, especially when combined with a large intake of water, can increase the filtering of the blood, washing it out, and in doing so even reduce its volume and lower blood pressure further. If your blood pressure is already naturally low, this can produce fatigue and dizziness if you get up quickly. People with low blood pressure should not go overboard with salt reduction and should limit their water intake to 1½ quarts per day.

On the other hand, too much salt leads to water retention. In hot climates, salt pills are regularly distributed to workers so that they avoid dehydration.

However many women, especially women intensely influenced by hormones during premenstrual or perimenopausal periods, or even during pregnancy, retain impressive amounts of water.

For these women, this water-reduction diet par excellence works most effectively when as little salt as possible is absorbed, allowing the water to pass more quickly through the body.

By the way, we often hear people complaining that they have put on 2 or even 4 pounds in one evening after a lapse in their diet. Sometimes a weight gain like this is not even due to a real lapse. When we analyze exactly what was eaten, we can never track down the 18,000 calories of food required to produce these 4 extra pounds. It was simply the combination of an oversalty meal accompanied by wine, beer, or cocktails. Salt and alcohol combine to slow down the elimination of the water drunk.

Never forget that 1 quart of water weighs 2 pounds, and 2 teaspoons of salt are enough to retain this water in your body's tissues for a day or two.

This being the case, if during your diet you cannot avoid a professional dinner engagement or family celebration that will force you to put aside the rules of the Dukan Diet, then at least avoid eating salty foods and drinking too much alcohol. And do not weigh yourself the next morning, because a sudden increase in weight may discourage you and undermine your determination and confidence. Wait until the following day—or, even better, for 2 days—while returning to the diet, drinking mineral water, with a low mineral content, and cutting back on salt. These three simple measures should be enough to get you back on track.

Salt increases appetite; decreasing your salt intake decreases your appetite. This is a simple observation. Salty foods increase salivation and gastric acidity, which in turn increase your appetite. Conversely, lightly salted foods have only a slight effect on digestive secretions and no effect on appetite. Unfortunately, the absence of salt reduces thirst, and when you follow the Dukan Diet, you have to accept that during the first days you will have to make yourself drink a large amount of liquid so that you boost your need for water and reestablish your natural thirst.

100
NATURAL FOODS
THAT KEEP YOU
SLIM

Eat As Much As You Like

MEAT

Beef tenderloin, filet mignon

Buffalo

Extra-lean ham

Extra-lean kosher beef hot dogs

Lean center-cut pork chops

Lean deli slices of roast beef

Pork tenderloin, pork loin roast

Reduced-fat bacon, soy bacon

Steak: flank, sirloin, London broil

Veal chops

Veal scaloppini

Venison

POULTRY

Chicken

Chicken liver

Cornish hen

Fat-free turkey and chicken sausage

Low-fat deli slices of chicken or turkey

Ostrich steak

Quail

Rabbit

Turkey

Wild duck

FISH

Arctic char

Catfish

Cod

Flounder

Grouper

Haddock

Halibut and smoked halibut

Herring

Mackerel

Mahi-mahi

Monkfish

Orange roughy

Perch

Red snapper

Salmon or smoked salmon

Sardines

Sea bass

Shark

Sole

Surimi

Swordfish

Tilapia

Trout

Tuna, fresh or canned in water

SHELLFISH
  Clams
  Crab
  Crawfish, crayfish
  Lobster
  Mussels
  Octopus
  Oysters
  Scallops
  Shrimp
  Squid

EGGS
  Chicken eggs

FAT-FREE DAIRY PRODUCTS
  Fat-free cottage cheese
  Fat-free cream cheese
  Fat-free milk
  Fat-free plain Greek-style yogurt, unsweetened or artificially sweetened
  Fat-free ricotta
  Fat-free sour cream

PLANT PROTEINS
  Seitan
  Soy foods and veggie burgers (pages 25–27)
  Tempeh
  Tofu

VEGETABLES
  Artichoke
  Asparagus
  Bean sprouts
  Beet
  Broccoli
  Brussels sprouts
  Cabbage

Carrots
Cauliflower
Celery
Cucumber
Eggplant
Endive
Fennel
Green beans
Kale
Lettuce, arugula, radicchio
Mushrooms
Okra
Onions, leeks, shallots
Palm hearts
Peppers
Pumpkin
Radishes
Rhubarb
Spaghetti squash
Spinach
Tomato
Turnip
Watercress
Zucchini

AND

Shirataki noodles
Sugar-free gelatin

THE
RECIPES

For a long time I thought that if I made the results the priority, people were bound to accept putting gastronomy and culinary delights on hold. I had not reckoned with my patients' and readers' ingenuity and unlimited creativity when they feel strongly motivated. They were amazingly inventive within the totally defined and structured framework that I had set for them, that of proteins and vegetables, but without any limits on quantity. Over the years, I have received thousands of recipes that use these foods and stick to the rules about how to prepare, combine, and alternate them. I have been amazed to see the extent to which people have been keen to share with others a recipe they really loved.

One day in 2005, I took a phone call from one of my readers who wanted to tell me that, having bought my book by chance in a train station, he had followed the instructions in it and by himself had lost more than 90 pounds in just over six months.

I have spent my life working as a chef. I love cooking just as much as I enjoy eating my food, so over the years I had become very overweight. Your program appealed to me because I'm a great fish and meat eater and, most important, I have a huge appetite, and your book starts off with the words "eat as much as you want."

I've drawn upon all my talent and expertise to bring the brilliance of great cooking to the foods that we are freely allowed and to the many recipes in your book. I have been having a feast for six months and I have lost weight without really suffering.

To thank you, I am going to send you these recipes from your repertoire, but which I have adapted for my own pleasure based on your rules, so that your readers and patients who lack time and imagination can enjoy them too.

Apart from being music to my ears, this phone call also struck a chord in my own family. My son, Sacha, who was studying nutrition, read these recipes and, together with this great and experienced chef, tested and created a range of diet dishes, all without any fat, flour, or sugar.

You will find these recipes in this book, along with other recipes, adaptations, and variations that are perhaps a little less professional, but every bit as creative, contributed by readers with a common goal of losing weight using my method and who post to Dukan Diet forums. I take this opportunity to thank, from the bottom of my heart, all those people who use the forums and have sent in their own versions of my recipes.

The Pure Protein Recipes

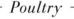 *Poultry*

Crispy Chicken Wings

MAKES 2 SERVINGS
Preparation time: 10 minutes, plus 2 to 3 hours for marinating
Cooking time: 10 minutes

¼ cup low-sodium soy sauce
1 garlic clove, crushed
2 teaspoons zero-calorie sweetener suited for cooking and
    baking, such as Splenda, dissolved in 1 teaspoon water
4 teaspoons five-spice powder (star anise, cloves, pepper,
    cinnamon, fennel)
1 teaspoon peeled and chopped fresh ginger
6 chicken wings, tips cut off (see Note)

1. In a medium dish, combine the soy sauce, garlic, sweetener, five-spice powder, and ginger.
2. Place the chicken wings in the dish and set in the refrigerator to marinate for 2 to 3 hours, turning them over once or twice.
3. Turn the oven on to Broil, and preheat for 5 minutes.
4. Place the chicken in a roasting pan. Cook under the broiler for 4 to 5 minutes, or until the wings start to hiss and crackle. Turn the wings over and cook for an additional 4 to 5 minutes, or until golden brown.
5. Remove the chicken from the oven and discard the skin before eating.

Note: The wing tips can be reserved and used for broth, see below and page 48.

Chicken Broth with Mussels

MAKES 6 SERVINGS
Preparation time: 30 minutes
Cooking time: 2 hours 5 minutes

3 pounds 5 ounces chicken wing tips
2 onions
2 shallots
1 head of garlic, cloves separated
4 stalks of celery
1 bouquet garni (make your own by tying together 6 sprigs of fresh parsley, 3 sprigs of fresh thyme, and 3 dried bay leaves)
Salt and freshly ground black pepper
2 pounds 4 ounces mussels
6 fresh chives, chopped
2 tablespoons chopped fresh parsley or chervil

1. Place 3 quarts of slightly salted water in a large pot and bring to a boil. Add the chicken wing tips, onions, shallots, garlic, celery, bouquet garni, and pepper to taste to the water.

2. Cover the pot and simmer for 2 hours over very low heat, taking care not to boil the broth (boiling will make the broth become cloudy).

3. Strain the cooked broth, bring to a boil, and add salt and pepper to taste.

4. Scrub and rinse the mussels several times. Discard any shells that are open or broken and that do not close when tapped.

5. Place the mussels in a large, high-sided frying pan with a lid, and add 1 cup of water.

6. Cook over high heat until the liquid comes to a boil. Reduce the heat to a simmer, cover the pot, and cook for about 3 minutes, until the mussels open. Discard any unopened mussels.

7. Strain the mussels and save the cooking juices. Shell the mussels, but leave a few unshelled in reserve to garnish the broth.

8. Divide the shelled mussels among six bowls, adding a little of the cooking juices.

9. To serve, pour the chicken broth over the mussels, sprinkle with the chopped herbs, and garnish with the unshelled mussels. Serve immediately.

Thai Chicken Broth

MAKES 2 SERVINGS
Preparation time: 10 minutes
Cooking time: 2 hours 30 minutes

2 chicken carcasses
1 onion, quartered
1 bunch of fresh cilantro, roughly chopped
2 fresh lemongrass stalks (white parts only), crushed
2 fresh kaffir lime leaves, chopped, or 2 teaspoons grated
    lime zest
1 tablespoon peeled and chopped fresh ginger
Salt and freshly ground black pepper

1. Put the chicken carcasses into a large pot and add 2 quarts of cold water. Bring to a boil, and with a ladle skim off and discard the scum that rises to the top.
2. Reduce the heat, and add the onion, cilantro, lemongrass, kaffir lime leaves or lime zest, and ginger to the pot. Cover and simmer over very low heat for 2½ hours, taking care not to boil (boiling will make the broth become cloudy). Strain the broth and add salt and pepper to taste before serving.

Note: Use the chicken bones and wing tips from other recipes, or some butchers will sell carcasses to you.

Mustardy Chicken Kebabs

MAKES 4 SERVINGS
Preparation time: 20 minutes, plus 2 hours for marinating
Cooking time: 15 minutes

4 boneless, skinless chicken breasts
1 low-sodium chicken bouillon cube
2 tablespoons Dijon mustard
1 teaspoon lemon juice
1 garlic clove, chopped
1 teaspoon cornstarch
¼ cup cold fat-free milk

1. Cut the chicken breasts into 1-inch chunks and put them in a large nonreactive bowl.
2. In a medium bowl, dissolve the bouillon cube in 1 cup of hot water.
3. Add the mustard, lemon juice, and garlic. Pour three-quarters of this marinade over the chicken, mix thoroughly, cover, and refrigerate for 2 hours.
4. Preheat oven to 425°F.
5. Thread the chicken chunks onto skewers (see Note) and place on a rack over a rimmed baking sheet. Roast them for about 7 minutes, or until just cooked through.

6. In a small saucepan, blend the cornstarch with the cold milk and add the remaining quarter of the marinade. Gently simmer the mixture over medium heat, stirring often, for 5 minutes, or until the sauce thickens. Serve alongside the kebabs.

Note: You will need 8 wooden or metal skewers for this recipe. If you are using wooden skewers, soak them in water for at least 30 minutes before using them so they won't burn.

Spicy Chicken Kebabs
MAKES 5 SERVINGS
Preparation time: 10 minutes, plus 2 to 3 hours for marinating
Cooking time: 10 minutes

1 cup fat-free plain Greek-style yogurt
1 teaspoon chili powder
1 teaspoon ground turmeric
1 teaspoon ground cumin
1 teaspoon ground coriander
1 teaspoon peeled and grated fresh ginger
1 garlic clove, crushed
2 pounds 4 ounces boneless, skinless chicken breasts, cut into
   1-inch cubes

1. In a medium bowl, combine the yogurt, chili, turmeric, cumin, coriander, ginger, and garlic.
2. Thread the chicken pieces onto skewers (see Note) and place in a dish big enough for the skewers to lie flat.
3. Cover the chicken with the marinade and place in the refrigerator, covered, for several hours or overnight.
4. When the chicken has marinated, heat up the barbecue or turn the oven on to Broil, and preheat for 5 minutes.
5. Place the kebabs under the broiler or on the barbecue and cook until the meat is browned and tender, about 8 minutes.

Note: You will need up to 25 small wooden or metal skewers for this recipe. If you are using wooden skewers, soak them in water for at least 30 minutes before using them so they won't burn.

Herb-Stuffed Chicken Legs

MAKES 2 SERVINGS
Preparation time: 10 minutes
Cooking time: 30 minutes

⅓ cup fat-free plain Greek-style yogurt
1 shallot, chopped
1 tablespoon chopped fresh parsley
20 fresh chives, finely chopped
Salt and freshly ground black pepper
2 chicken legs with thighs attached, skin removed

1. Preheat oven to 375°F.
2. In a medium bowl, combine the yogurt, shallot, parsley, and chives. Season with salt and pepper to taste.
3. Using a sharp, pointed knife, make an incision into the thickest part of each chicken thigh, about 1½ inches long and 1 inch deep.
4. Push the yogurt mixture into the slits and coat the chicken thighs with the rest of the mixture.
5. Cut out two 8 × 8-inch sheets of aluminum foil and place a chicken thigh in the center of each piece, closing the foil to form a parcel.
6. Put a little water in the bottom of a small baking dish and place the parcels in it.
7. Bake in the oven for 30 minutes.

Tandoori Chicken

MAKES 6 SERVINGS

Preparation time: 15 minutes, plus overnight marinating

Cooking time: 10 minutes

6 boneless, skinless chicken breasts

3 garlic cloves, crushed

2 teaspoons peeled and very finely chopped fresh ginger

2 fresh green chili peppers, very finely chopped

1 cup fat-free plain Greek-style yogurt

2 teaspoons tandoori masala spice mix

Juice of 1 lemon

Salt and freshly ground black pepper

1. Put each chicken breast on a sheet of plastic wrap and beat with a rolling pin until ¼ inch thick.
2. In a medium nonreactive bowl, mix together the garlic, ginger, chilies, yogurt, tandoori masala, and lemon juice until thoroughly combined. Add salt and pepper to taste.
3. Make several ⅛-inch-deep incisions into each chicken breast. Place the chicken in a glass baking dish and thoroughly coat with the yogurt mixture. Cover and refrigerate overnight.
4. The following day, preheat the oven to 400°F.
5. Cook the chicken for 5 minutes, then turn the oven temperature up to Broil and cook for an additional 2 minutes, or until brown.

Barbecued Curry Chicken

MAKES 4 SERVINGS

Preparation time: 5 minutes, plus 2 hours for marinating

Cooking time: 5 minutes

4 boneless, skinless chicken breasts

1 cup fat-free plain Greek-style yogurt

1 tablespoon curry powder

Salt and freshly ground black pepper

1. Put each chicken breast on a sheet of plastic wrap and beat with a rolling pin until ¼ inch thick.
2. In a small bowl, mix together the yogurt and curry powder, and add salt and pepper to taste.
3. Place the chicken in a glass baking dish and thoroughly coat with the yogurt mixture. Cover with plastic wrap and allow the chicken to marinate for 2 hours in the refrigerator.
4. When the chicken has marinated, heat up the barbecue or turn the oven on to Broil and preheat for 5 minutes.
5. Barbecue or broil the chicken pieces for 5 minutes, turning once.

Lemongrass Chicken

MAKES 8 SERVINGS
Preparation time: 30 minutes
Cooking time: 20 minutes

⅛ teaspoon vegetable oil
3 pounds 5 ounces boneless, skinless chicken breasts, cut into ¼-inch strips
2 small onions, finely chopped
3 fresh lemongrass stalks, white parts only, finely chopped
A pinch of chili powder
2 tablespoons nuoc mam (Vietnamese fish sauce)
2 tablespoons low-sodium soy sauce
2 tablespoons zero-calorie sweetener suited for cooking and baking, such as Splenda
Salt and freshly ground black pepper

1. Heat a large, heavy-bottomed skillet over medium heat. Add the oil and wipe out any excess with a paper towel.
2. Add the chicken and cook, stirring often, until brown.
3. Add the onions, lemongrass, chili powder, nuoc mam, soy sauce, sweetener, and salt and pepper to taste.
4. Lower the heat, cover the pan, and cook for 15 minutes.

Marinated Indian Chicken

MAKES 4 SERVINGS

Preparation time: 40 minutes, plus 24 hours for marinating
Cooking time: 40 minutes

2 cups fat-free plain Greek-style yogurt
¼ cup peeled and chopped fresh ginger
3 garlic cloves, chopped
1 teaspoon cinnamon
2 pinches of cayenne pepper
1 teaspoon coriander seeds
3 cloves
Grated zest of 1 lemon
10 fresh mint leaves, chopped
1 whole chicken, about 3 pounds, quartered and skin removed
Salt and freshly ground black pepper
2 onions, chopped

1. In a medium bowl, mix together the yogurt, ginger, garlic, cinnamon, cayenne, coriander, cloves, lemon zest, and mint leaves.
2. Season the chicken pieces with salt and pepper to taste and coat with the yogurt mixture.
3. Cover the bowl and refrigerate for 24 hours.
4. Place a nonstick, heatproof casserole over medium heat, add 1 tablespoon of water and the chopped onions, and cook until browned.
5. Add the chicken and the marinade. Cover and bring to a simmer, then cook over gentle heat for about 40 minutes, or until a thermometer inserted into the thickest part of the chicken registers 170°F.
6. Serve piping hot.

Note: The leftover juices can be made into a soup with the addition of low-sodium chicken stock or a low-sodium chicken bouillon cube and water.

Ginger Chicken

MAKES 4 SERVINGS

Preparation time: 20 minutes

Cooking time: 1 hour 10 minutes

⅛ teaspoon vegetable oil

2 large onions, finely chopped

3 garlic cloves, finely chopped

8 cloves

1 whole chicken, about 3 pounds, quartered and skin removed

1 tablespoon peeled and grated fresh ginger

Salt and freshly ground black pepper

1. Heat a large, heavy-bottomed skillet over medium heat. Add the oil and wipe out any excess with a paper towel.
2. Add the onions and the garlic and cook, stirring often, until browned.
3. Stick cloves into the chicken pieces and add to the skillet.
4. Add enough water to cover the chicken halfway. Add the ginger and season with salt and pepper to taste.
5. Cover and cook over medium heat for about 1 hour, or until a thermometer inserted into the thickest part of the chicken registers 170°F and nearly all the water has evaporated.

Thyme Chicken with Herb Sauce

MAKES 4 SERVINGS

Preparation time: 35 minutes

Cooking time: 25 minutes

1 bunch of fresh thyme

1 whole chicken, about 3 pounds, quartered and skin removed

Salt and freshly ground black pepper

2 shallots, finely chopped

2 cups fat-free plain Greek-style yogurt

Juice of 1 lemon

1 bunch of fresh parsley, finely chopped

1 tablespoon chopped fresh mint leaves

1 garlic clove, finely chopped

1. Fill the bottom part of a large steamer with water and bring to a boil.
2. In the upper part of the steamer, spread out half the thyme sprigs, place the chicken pieces on top of them, and season to taste with salt and pepper. Cover with the rest of the thyme sprigs and the chopped shallots.
3. Put the lid on the steamer and as soon as steam starts to escape, cook for 20 to 25 minutes, or until a thermometer inserted into the thickest part of the chicken registers 170°F.
4. While the chicken is cooking, pour the yogurt into a medium nonreactive bowl, and add the lemon juice, parsley, mint leaves, and garlic. Add salt and pepper to taste, then mix all the ingredients together thoroughly, cover, and refrigerate.
5. Serve the yogurt sauce as an accompaniment for the chicken.

Note: You will need a large steamer for this recipe.

Easy Chicken Curry

MAKES 4 SERVINGS
Preparation time: 15 minutes
Cooking time: 45 minutes

⅛ teaspoon vegetable oil
1 whole chicken, about 3 pounds, quartered and skin removed
½ cup chopped onions
1 cup fat-free plain Greek-style yogurt
1 teaspoon ground ginger
1 teaspoon paprika
Grated zest of 1 lemon
2 teaspoons lemon juice
2 teaspoons curry powder
Salt and freshly ground black pepper

1. Heat a nonstick frying pan. Add the oil and wipe out any excess with a paper towel.
2. Place the chicken pieces in a nonstick frying pan.
3. Mix the onions, yogurt, ginger, paprika, lemon zest, lemon juice, and curry powder together, then pour over the chicken and cover the pan.
4. Place the pan over medium heat and bring to a simmer. Reduce the heat, cover, and continue simmering for 45 minutes, or until a thermometer inserted into the thickest part of the chicken registers 170°F.
5. Season with salt and pepper to taste.
6. Uncover the pan and cook until the sauce is thickened.

Chicken with Lemons

MAKES 2 TO 3 SERVINGS
Preparation time: 15 minutes
Cooking time: 30 minutes

⅛ teaspoon vegetable oil

1 onion, finely chopped

2 garlic cloves, finely chopped

1 teaspoon peeled and finely chopped fresh ginger

1 pound boneless, skinless chicken breasts, cut into
    1-inch cubes

Grated zest and juice of 2 lemons

2 tablespoons low-sodium soy sauce

1 bouquet garni (make your own by tying together 6 sprigs
    of fresh parsley, 3 sprigs of fresh thyme, and 3 dried bay
    leaves)

A pinch of ground cinnamon

A pinch of ground ginger

Salt and freshly ground black pepper

1. Heat a deep nonstick skillet over medium heat. Add the oil and wipe out any excess with a paper towel.

2. Add the onion, garlic, and fresh ginger and cook for 3 to 4 minutes, or until browned.

3. Increase the heat to high, add the chicken, and sauté for 2 minutes, stirring constantly.

4. Add the lemon zest, lemon juice, soy sauce, ⅔ cup of water, and the bouquet garni, cinnamon, and ground ginger. Add salt and pepper to taste.

5. Reduce the heat to a gentle simmer, cover, and cook for 20 minutes.

Cardamom Chicken

MAKES 4 SERVINGS

Preparation time: 20 minutes

Cooking time: 30 minutes

⅛ teaspoon vegetable oil

4 chicken thighs, skin removed

2 garlic cloves, finely chopped

2 onions, finely chopped

A pinch of five-spice powder (star anise, cloves, pepper, cinnamon, fennel)

2 teaspoons curry powder

2 cups fat-free plain Greek-style yogurt

1 cinnamon stick

2 teaspoons ground cumin

10 cardamom pods

A pinch of saffron threads

A pinch of cayenne pepper

1. Heat a deep nonstick skillet over medium heat. Add the oil and wipe out any excess with a paper towel.
2. Add the chicken thighs and cook until browned. Turn the chicken over and brown the other side.
3. Add the garlic and onions and cook for an additional 4 minutes.
4. In a medium bowl, combine the five-spice powder, curry powder, and yogurt. Pour the yogurt mixture over the chicken.
5. Cover, reduce the heat, and simmer for 10 minutes.
6. Add the cinnamon stick, cumin, cardamom, saffron, and cayenne. Cover and continue cooking for an additional 10 minutes.
7. Place the chicken thighs on a heated serving dish. Strain the sauce and process in a blender for a few seconds, until it is completely smooth. Pour the sauce over the chicken and serve immediately.

Chicken Rillettes

MAKES 3 SERVINGS

Preparation time: 15 minutes, plus 2 hours for refrigeration

Cooking time: 5 minutes

⅛ teaspoon vegetable oil

1 pound boneless, skinless chicken or turkey breast, cut into
   ½-inch cubes

2 onions, roughly chopped

5 gherkin pickles*

½ cup fat-free plain Greek-style yogurt

A pinch of chili powder

A pinch of ground or grated nutmeg

Salt and freshly ground black pepper

1. Heat a heavy-bottomed frying pan over high heat. Add the oil and wipe out any excess with a paper towel.
2. Add the chicken pieces and cook, stirring often, for 5 minutes, or until brown.
3. Place the chicken pieces, onions, gherkins, yogurt, chili powder, and nutmeg in a food processor and blend, pulsing on and off, until the texture is smooth, but still thick and somewhat textured. Add salt and pepper to taste.
4. Place the chicken mixture into a loaf pan, packing it tightly. Cover and refrigerate for at least 2 hours before serving.

Note: You will need a loaf pan for this recipe.

*Use only no-sugar-added pickles.

Sautéed Chicken with Lemon and Capers

MAKES 4 SERVINGS
Preparation time: 20 minutes
Cooking time: 15 minutes

⅛ teaspoon vegetable oil
1 small red onion, finely chopped
1½ pounds boneless, skinless chicken breasts, cut into thin
    slices across the grain of the meat
Grated zest of 1 lemon
1 tablespoon small capers, drained and rinsed
1 tablespoon fresh lemon juice
5 fresh basil leaves, finely chopped
Salt and freshly ground black pepper

1. Heat a nonstick, heavy-bottomed frying pan over medium heat. Add the oil and wipe out any excess with a paper towel.
2. Add the onion and cook, stirring often, until it turns golden brown. Remove from the pan and reserve.
3. Add the chicken slices to the same pan and cook, stirring often, until browned, about 7 minutes.
4. Add the reserved onion, lemon zest, capers, lemon juice, and basil, and stir thoroughly. Add salt and pepper to taste.

Chicken and Parsley Terrine

MAKES 8 SERVINGS
Preparation time: 40 minutes, plus 2 hours 20 minutes for refrigeration
Cooking time: 15 minutes

2 (7-gram) envelopes of unflavored gelatin
1 large bunch of fresh parsley, stems removed, finely
    chopped
7 ounces cooked boneless, skinless chicken or turkey, diced

1. In a small saucepan, mix the gelatin and 2 cups plus 1 tablespoon of cold water. Bring the mixture to a boil slowly,

stirring constantly. As soon as the first bubbles appear, remove the pan from the heat and leave to cool.

2. Pour a thin layer of the gelatin into a loaf pan, cover, and put into the freezer for 3 minutes.

3. Combine the remaining gelatin mixture with the parsley and chicken.

4. Pour half of the chicken mixture into the loaf pan, cover, and freeze for 15 minutes.

5. Add the rest of the mixture to the loaf pan, cover, and refrigerate for 2 hours.

6. To turn the terrine out of the loaf pan, immerse the bottom of the pan into some hot water, then invert the loaf pan onto a large plate. The terrine will slide out.

Note: You will need a loaf pan for this recipe.

Chicken Sauté with Chilies

MAKES 4 SERVINGS

Preparation time: 35 minutes

Cooking time: 10 minutes

6 small red onions or shallots

3 to 6 fresh red chilies

1-inch piece of fresh ginger, peeled

1 fresh lemongrass stalk

4 garlic cloves

⅛ teaspoon vegetable oil

4 boneless, skinless chicken breasts, each cut long ways into 8 strips

Salt and freshly ground black pepper

1. Cut one onion into thin slices to garnish the dish. In a blender, combine the chilies, half the ginger, and the lemongrass until puréed. Remove the chili mixture from the blender and reserve.

2. In the blender, combine the remaining onions, the garlic, and the remaining half of the ginger and purée.
3. Heat a large nonstick frying pan over medium heat. Add the oil and wipe out any excess with a paper towel.
4. Add the chili purée and cook for 2 minutes, stirring constantly.
5. Add the chicken pieces and stir until they are well covered with the chili purée.
6. Add ⅔ cup water and the onion purée to the chicken mixture, and stir until combined. Add salt and pepper to taste.
7. Cook, uncovered, over high heat for 5 minutes.
8. Serve hot, garnished with the raw onion slices.

Chicken Liver and Parsley Soufflé

MAKES 4 SERVINGS
Preparation time: 20 minutes
Cooking time: 35 minutes

⅛ teaspoon vegetable oil
9 ounces chicken livers
1 garlic clove
1 bunch of fresh parsley
4 eggs, separated
2 cups plus 2 tablespoons Béchamel Sauce (page 344)
Salt and freshly ground black pepper

1. Preheat oven to 350°F.
2. Heat a nonstick frying pan over medium heat. Add the oil and wipe out any excess with a paper towel.
3. Add the chicken livers and cook until browned.
4. Remove them from the pan and place on a cutting board with the garlic and parsley. Chop the livers, garlic, and parsley.
5. In a medium bowl, combine the chopped liver mixture, egg yolks, and béchamel sauce. Season with salt and pepper to taste.

6. In an electric mixer, beat the egg whites until stiff, then gently fold them into the liver mixture.

7. Pour the mixture into a 1½-quart soufflé dish and bake for 30 minutes, or until a deep golden brown. Serve immediately.

Chicken Liver and Tarragon Terrine

MAKES 4 SERVINGS

Preparation time: 15 minutes, plus overnight refrigeration

Cooking time: 5 minutes

⅛ teaspoon vegetable oil

10 ounces chicken livers

3 tablespoons raspberry vinegar

1 bunch of fresh tarragon, stems removed

½ cup fat-free plain Greek-style yogurt

Salt and freshly ground black pepper

1. Heat a large nonstick frying pan over high heat. Add the oil and wipe out any excess with a paper towel.

2. Add the chicken livers and cook until browned, stirring often.

3. Remove the livers from the pan and place in a blender.

4. Add the vinegar to the hot pan and stir to deglaze.

5. To the livers in the blender add the vinegar, tarragon leaves, yogurt, and salt and pepper to taste .

6. Purée the ingredients in the blender, then pour the mixture into a loaf pan.

7. Cover and refrigerate overnight before serving.

8. To turn the terrine out of the pan, immerse the bottom of the pan in some hot water then invert it onto a large plate. The terrine will slide out. Slice and serve.

Note: You will need a loaf pan for this recipe.

Lime and Salt–Crusted Cornish Game Hen

MAKES 2 SERVINGS

Preparation time: 25 minutes, plus overnight marinating

Cooking time: 30 minutes

1 bouquet garni (make your own by tying together 6 sprigs
of fresh parsley, 3 sprigs of fresh thyme, and 3 dried bay
leaves)

Juice of 1 lime

1 onion, chopped

1 Cornish game hen, about 1 pound

2 egg whites

1 cup coarse sea salt

Salt and freshly ground black pepper

1. A day in advance of cooking, put the bouquet garni, half the lime juice, the onion, and the Cornish game hen into a large, nonreactive container. Add 5 cups of cold water, cover, and refrigerate overnight.
2. When ready to cook, preheat the oven to 425°F.
3. Strain the marinade and discard the liquid; reserve the onion and bouquet garni. Stuff the reserved solids from the marinade into the cavity of the bird.
4. Mix the egg whites with the sea salt and cover the bottom of a baking dish with about half the salt mixture.
5. Place the hen in the middle of the baking dish and cover it with the remaining salt mixture.
6. Roast for 30 minutes, or until a thermometer inserted into the thickest part of the thigh registers 170°F.
7. To serve, break the salt crust with the back of a spoon, brush away the salt, and carefully remove the skin. Halve the hen and drizzle the remaining lime juice over it before serving.
8. Season with salt and pepper to taste.

Turkey and Bresaola Parcels

MAKES 4 SERVINGS
Preparation time: 15 minutes
Cooking time: 30 minutes

4 pieces of boneless, skinless turkey breasts, approximately
    5 ounces each
4 tablespoons mustard
4 slices of bresaola (see Note)
1 tablespoon herbes de Provence (a mix of dried marjoram,
    thyme, savory, basil, rosemary, sage, and fennel seeds)
Salt and freshly ground black pepper

1. Preheat oven to 350°F.
2. Remove any fat from the turkey breasts, then place each one on a square of aluminum foil.
3. Coat each turkey breast with 1 tablespoon of mustard, wrap a slice of bresaola around the breast, and sprinkle with the herbes de Provence. Add salt and pepper to taste.
4. Sprinkle ¼ teaspoon of water over each turkey breast, seal up the foil parcels, place on a baking sheet, and bake in the oven for 30 minutes.

Note: If bresaola is not available, you may substitute turkey bacon.

Nutmeg and Milk–Braised Turkey

MAKES 4 SERVINGS
Preparation time: 20 minutes
Cooking time: 1 hour

1 whole boneless turkey breast, about 2¼ pounds
Salt and freshly ground black pepper
A pinch of ground nutmeg
5 garlic cloves
4 cups fat-free milk

1. Preheat oven to 425°F.
2. Season the turkey with salt and pepper to taste and the nutmeg.
3. Place the turkey and garlic in a deep nonstick, heatproof casserole or a small Dutch oven, and pour the milk over the turkey. If the casserole is the correct size, at least three-quarters of the turkey will be submerged in the milk. Add more milk if the turkey isn't three-quarters submerged.
4. Over medium heat, warm the casserole for about 5 minutes on the top of the stove, then place in the oven and bake for 40 minutes, or until a thermometer inserted into the thickest part of the turkey registers 170°F. Turn the bird over every 10 minutes for even cooking.
5. After the turkey has reached 170°F, turn off the oven, cover the dish, and leave it in the hot oven for an additional 10 minutes.
6. Remove the dish from the oven, strain the sauce, and reserve.
7. Remove the skin from the turkey, carve, and serve with the strained sauce.

Pink Peppercorn Turkey Cutlets

MAKES 4 SERVINGS
Preparation time: 20 minutes
Cooking time: 20 minutes

4 pieces boneless, skinless turkey breasts, approximately
    5 ounces each
⅓ cup fat-free plain Greek-style yogurt
1 teaspoon cornstarch
2 teaspoons whole-grain mustard
2 teaspoons Dijon mustard
Salt and freshly ground black pepper
2 teaspoons ground pink peppercorns
2 sprigs of fresh thyme, chopped (about ¼ teaspoon)

1. Preheat oven to 350°F.
2. Put each turkey breast on a sheet of plastic wrap and beat with a rolling pin until ¼ inch thick.

3. Heat a large nonstick frying pan over medium heat. Place the turkey in the pan and cook for 1 minute on each side. Place the turkey on a plate and reserve.

4. In a small bowl, combine the yogurt, cornstarch, and whole-grain and Dijon mustards. Season the mustard mixture with salt and pepper to taste and the pink peppercorns.

5. Cut out four 8 × 12-inch rectangles of parchment paper. Place a piece of turkey on each sheet, then place a quarter of the sauce on top of each turkey piece. Sprinkle the thyme on top.

6. Close the parcels up by folding the parchment paper over on itself several times.

7. Place the parcels in a large ovenproof dish and bake in the oven for 15 minutes.

Turkey Meat Loaf

MAKES 4 SERVINGS
Preparation time: 15 minutes
Cooking time: 30 minutes

1 pound ground turkey or chicken
1 large onion, finely chopped
2 tablespoons mixed dried herbs and spices, such as cumin
    seeds, basil, herbes de Provence, paprika, and ginger
Salt and freshly ground black pepper
6 eggs
2 tablespoons cornstarch
⅛ teaspoon vegetable oil

1. Preheat oven to 350°F.

2. In a large bowl, combine the turkey and onion. Add the herbs and spices, along with salt and pepper to taste.

3. In a medium bowl, lightly beat the eggs. Add the cornstarch, and whisk to combine.

4. Add the eggs to the turkey mixture and stir to combine.

5. Add oil to a 9-inch nonstick square cake pan or medium gratin dish and wipe out any excess with a paper towel. Bake for 25 minutes.

6. Remove the dish from the oven and gently run a knife around the edge of the pan. Turn the meat loaf out onto a serving dish or cutting board. Slice and serve.

Turkey Timbales

MAKES 2 SERVINGS
Preparation time: 30 minutes
Cooking time: 20 minutes

3 tablespoons fat-free plain Greek-style yogurt
1 shallot, chopped
1 tablespoon fresh parsley, finely chopped
1 garlic clove, crushed
1 tablespoon fresh lemon juice
Salt and freshly ground black pepper
⅛ teaspoon vegetable oil
9 ounces boneless, skinless turkey breast, cut into very
    thin strips

1. Preheat oven to 350°F.
2. In a nonreactive medium bowl, mix together the yogurt, shallot, parsley, garlic, and lemon juice. Add salt and pepper to taste.
3. Lightly coat two 2-cup ramekins with the vegetable oil and wipe out the excess.
4. In the prepared ramekins, alternate layers of turkey strips with the herb mixture, finishing off with a layer of turkey.
5. Place the ramekins into a large baking dish and fill the large dish half full with cold water.
6. Place the large baking dish in the oven and cook the timbales until are set, about 20 minutes.

7. Carefully remove the baking dish from the oven, and the ramekins from the hot water. Gently run a knife around the edge of the ramekins. Turn out each timbale onto a serving dish and serve hot.

Note: You will need two 2-cup ramekins for this recipe.

--- *Meat* ---

Vietnamese Beef

MAKES 2 SERVINGS
Preparation time: 10 minutes, plus 30 minutes for marinating
Cooking time: 5 minutes

10 ounces sirloin steak
2 tablespoons low-sodium soy sauce
1 tablespoon oyster sauce
1 tablespoon peeled and crushed fresh ginger
Freshly ground black pepper
⅛ teaspoon vegetable oil
4 garlic cloves, crushed
A few fresh cilantro leaves, chopped

1. Cut the steak into ½-inch cubes.
2. In a small bowl, mix together the soy sauce, oyster sauce, and ginger, and add pepper to taste.
3. Put the meat into a dish and pour the soy sauce mixture over it.
4. Cover the meat and marinate in the refrigerator for at least 30 minutes.
5. Heat a medium, heavy-bottomed skillet over medium heat, add the oil and wipe out any excess with a paper towel.
6. Add the garlic and cook, stirring often, until just browned.
7. While the garlic is cooking, remove the meat from the marinade and drain. Add the meat to the browned garlic in the skillet.

8. Increase the heat to high and cook, stirring rapidly, for 10 to 15 seconds. The meat should be served on the rare side, so do not overcook it.

9. Garnish with cilantro leaves and serve.

Meatballs with Rosemary and Mint

MAKES 4 SERVINGS

Preparation time: 15 minutes

Cooking time: 20 minutes

1 medium onion, chopped

1½ pounds 95% lean ground beef

2 garlic cloves, crushed

1 egg, lightly beaten

2 tablespoons sugar-free ketchup or water

1 tablespoon Worcestershire sauce

2 tablespoons finely chopped fresh rosemary

1 to 2 tablespoons finely chopped fresh mint or basil

Salt and freshly ground black pepper

⅛ teaspoon vegetable oil

1. In a large bowl, mix together the onion, ground beef, garlic, egg, ketchup or water, Worcestershire, and the rosemary and mint or basil. Add salt and pepper to taste, and shape the mixture into meatballs the size of a walnut.

2. Heat a large nonstick skillet over medium-high heat. Add the oil and wipe out any excess with a paper towel.

3. Cook the meatballs, a few at a time, turning while cooking, until they are golden brown on all sides, about 5 minutes.

4. Place the cooked meatballs on a plate lined with a paper towel to absorb any fat before serving.

Asian Meatballs

MAKES 4 SERVINGS

Preparation time: 20 minutes

Cooking time: 30 minutes

1 pound lean ground veal or lean ground beef

⅛ teaspoon vegetable oil

3 tablespoons low-sodium soy sauce

2 tablespoons sherry vinegar

1 low-sodium beef bouillon cube

2 large garlic cloves, finely chopped

1 teaspoon peeled and grated fresh ginger

2 shallots, finely chopped

Salt and freshly ground black pepper

1 teaspoon cornstarch

1. Shape the veal or ground beef into small meatballs the size of a walnut.
2. Heat a large nonstick skillet over high heat. Add the oil and wipe out any excess with a paper towel.
3. Cook the meatballs, a few at a time, turning while cooking, until they are golden brown on all sides, about 5 minutes. Place the cooked meatballs on a plate lined with a paper towel to absorb any fat.
4. Pour a cup of water into the pan and mix it thoroughly with the meat juices. Add the soy sauce, vinegar, bouillon, garlic, ginger, and shallots, along with salt and pepper to taste. Mix until well combined and the bouillon is dissolved.
5. Return the meatballs to the pan, adding enough water to cover the meatballs halfway in sauce.
6. Cook over medium heat for 10 minutes, turning the meatballs a few times.
7. Remove the meatballs and place on a serving platter.
8. In a small bowl, combine the cornstarch with 1 tablespoon of cold water and mix until no lumps remain.
9. Add the cornstarch to the sauce, whisk to combine, and heat thoroughly. Pour sauce over meatballs and serve.

Calf's Liver with Raspberry Vinegar

MAKES 1 SERVING
Preparation time: 15 minutes
Cooking time: 20 minutes

⅛ teaspoon vegetable oil
1 small onion, thinly sliced
3 ounces calf's liver, sliced into ¼-inch slices
Salt and freshly ground black pepper
1 shallot, finely chopped
1 tablespoon raspberry vinegar
1 teaspoon dried thyme
1 dried bay leaf

1. Heat a heavy-bottomed skillet over medium heat. Add the oil and wipe out any excess with a paper towel.
2. Add the onion and cook until golden brown. Remove the cooked onion from the skillet and reserve on a plate.
3. Place the calf's liver in the hot skillet and cook for about 3 minutes on each side. The insides of the slices should still be pink.
4. Season the liver with salt and pepper to taste, place on the plate with the onions, and cover.
5. Add the shallot to the hot pan and cook until soft.
6. Add the raspberry vinegar, thyme, and bay leaf to the shallot and cook for an additional 2 minutes, stirring constantly.
7. Place the liver and onions back in the frying pan and heat the mixture through, taking care not to overcook the liver. Remove the bay leaf before serving.

Ham Roulades

MAKES 4 SERVINGS

Preparation time: 10 minutes, plus 30 minutes for refrigeration

Cooking time: No cooking required

1 garlic clove, finely chopped
1 bunch of fresh chives, chopped
¾ cup fat-free ricotta
8 slices of extra-lean ham
4 sprigs of fresh parsley

1. In a medium bowl, combine the garlic, chives, and ricotta.
2. Spread the ricotta mixture over the slices of ham and roll them up.
3. Place the rolls on a plate, cover with plastic wrap, and refrigerate for 30 minutes.
4. To serve, place 2 ham rolls on each plate, and garnish with a sprig of parsley.

Ham Bites

MAKES 2 SERVINGS

Preparation time: 10 minutes

Cooking time: No cooking required

6 ounces extra-lean ham, chopped
¾ cup fat-free ricotta
3 fresh chives, finely chopped
2 shallots, finely chopped
¼ teaspoon finely chopped fresh marjoram or fresh oregano
Tabasco sauce

1. In a large bowl, combine ham, ricotta, chives, shallots, the marjoram or oregano, and Tabasco.
2. Roll the mixture into tiny balls about ¼ inch in diameter.
3. Place balls on a plate, cover with plastic wrap, and chill until ready to serve.

Country Pâté

MAKES 8 SERVINGS
Preparation time: 20 minutes
Cooking time: 1 hour

12 ounces sliced deli turkey
7 ounces chicken livers
9 ounces extra-lean ham
1 onion, quartered
1 pound 9 ounces 95% lean ground beef
⅛ teaspoon ground cloves
4 garlic cloves, crushed
1 tablespoon port, boiled
1 pinch of ground nutmeg
1 teaspoon dried thyme
1 teaspoon dried oregano
Freshly ground black pepper

1. Preheat oven to 400°F.
2. In a food processor, finely chop a third of the turkey with all of the chicken livers, ham, and onion.
3. Place the mixture into a large bowl and add the ground beef.
4. In a small bowl, combine the cloves, garlic, port, nutmeg, thyme, and oregano, along with pepper to taste. Mix the seasonings into the meat mixture.
5. Line a 9-inch loaf pan with the remaining turkey slices so that they generously overlap the sides of the pan. (You will use the overlap to cover the filled loaf pan.)
6. Firmly press the mixture into the loaf pan, then tap the pan on a hard surface to get rid of any air bubbles.
7. Fold the turkey over the top, cover with aluminum foil, and bake for 1 hour.
8. Allow the pâté to cool for 5 minutes, drain off any surplus liquid, and let cool completely, uncovered.
9. To serve, invert pâté onto a plate and slice with a serrated knife.

Note: You will need a 9-inch loaf pan for this recipe.

Herbed Chicken and Rabbit Bundles

MAKES 4 SERVINGS

Preparation time: 15 minutes

Cooking time: 35 minutes

2 boneless, skinless chicken breasts

⅛ teaspoon vegetable oil

2 boneless saddles of rabbit

1 teaspoon mixed dried herbs, such as thyme, bay leaves,
savory, and marjoram or rosemary

Salt and freshly ground black pepper

1. Preheat oven to 425°F.
2. Put each chicken breast on a sheet of plastic wrap and beat with a rolling pin until ¼ inch thick.
3. Heat a nonstick skillet over high heat. Add the oil and wipe out any excess with a paper towel.
4. Add the chicken and cook quickly, about 1 minute on each side. Cut each breast in half.
5. Cut each rabbit saddle into two pieces. Wrap half a chicken breast around each piece and secure with butcher's twine.
6. Place each bundle on an 8 × 8-inch square of aluminum foil. Sprinkle each bundle with a quarter of the herbs, and season with salt and pepper to taste.
7. Close the foil around each bundle and bake on a baking sheet for 30 minutes. Remove the butcher's twine before serving.

Rabbit in a Mustard and Caper Sauce

MAKES 4 SERVINGS

Preparation time: 30 minutes

Cooking time: 35 minutes

⅛ teaspoon vegetable oil

1 rabbit, cut into pieces (see Note)

1 shallot, finely chopped

Salt and freshly ground black pepper

3 tablespoons fat-free plain Greek-style yogurt

1 tablespoon mustard

1 tablespoon capers, drained and rinsed

3 gherkin pickles,* sliced

1. Preheat oven to 375°F.
2. Heat a large, ovenproof heavy-bottomed skillet over medium heat. Add the oil and wipe out any excess with a paper towel.
3. Add the rabbit and shallot and cook until browned on both sides, about 4 minutes per side.
4. Season the rabbit with salt and pepper to taste and place the skillet in the oven.
5. Cook for 20 minutes, or until a thermometer inserted into the thickest part of the rabbit registers 160°F.
6. Remove the skillet from the oven and mix in the yogurt, mustard, capers, and gherkin pickles.
7. Place the skillet on the stove and heat for a couple of minutes over medium heat until hot, being careful not to allow the sauce to boil.

Note: You can substitute a 3- to 3½-pound chicken for the rabbit.

*Use only no-sugar-added pickles.

Eggs

Smoked Salmon with Scrambled Eggs

MAKES 4 SERVINGS
Preparation time: 10 minutes
Cooking time: 10 minutes

8 eggs
Salt and freshly ground black pepper
¼ cup fat-free milk
3 ounces smoked salmon, cut into thin strips
1 tablespoon fat-free ricotta
4 fresh chives, chopped

1. In a medium bowl, beat the eggs and season with salt and pepper to taste.
2. Pour the milk into a medium heavy-bottomed pan and warm over medium heat. Pour in the eggs and cook, stirring continuously with a spatula.
3. Remove the pan from the heat and stir in the salmon and ricotta.
4. Decorate the salmon and eggs with chives before serving.

Scrambled Eggs with Herbs

MAKES 2 SERVINGS
Preparation time: 10 minutes
Cooking time: 10 minutes

4 eggs
½ cup fat-free milk
Salt and freshly ground black pepper
A pinch of ground nutmeg
2 sprigs of fresh parsley or 4 fresh chives, chopped

1. In a medium heatproof glass bowl, beat the eggs thoroughly. Add the milk and season with salt and pepper to taste. Add the nutmeg.
2. Fill a medium pot with water and bring to a simmer.
3. Place the bowl over the pot. The bottom of the bowl should not touch the water. Stirring constantly, cook the eggs until they are creamy and barely set.
4. Sprinkle the eggs with the chopped parsley or chives and serve.

Scrambled Eggs with Crab

MAKES 3 SERVINGS
Preparation time: 10 minutes
Cooking time: 10 minutes

6 medium eggs
2 tablespoons nuoc mam (Vietnamese fish sauce)
⅛ teaspoon vegetable oil
2 medium shallots, finely chopped
3 ounces white crabmeat, well drained

1. In a medium bowl, lightly beat together the eggs and the nuoc mam.
2. Heat a medium nonstick skillet over medium heat. Add the oil and wipe out any excess with a paper towel.
3. Add the shallots and cook until they turn golden, about 1 minute.
4. Remove the shallots from the skillet and add to the eggs.
5. Cook the crabmeat in the skillet until it is slightly browned, stirring continuously, for about 3 minutes.
6. Add the eggs and cook for about 3 minutes, until the eggs are just scrambled but not browned.

Eggs Cocotte with Smoked Salmon

MAKES 6 SERVINGS
Preparation time: 10 minutes
Cooking time: 5 minutes

⅛ teaspoon vegetable oil
¼ cup fat-free ricotta
2 teaspoons chopped fresh tarragon or fresh chervil
3 ounces smoked salmon, cut into thin strips
6 eggs
Salt and freshly ground black pepper

1. Divide the oil evenly among six 1-cup ramekins and wipe out excess with a paper towel.
2. Place 2 teaspoons of the ricotta and a pinch of the herbs into each ramekin.
3. Evenly distribute the salmon among the ramekins. Crack 1 egg over the salmon in each ramekin. Season with salt and pepper to taste.
4. In a high-sided saucepan large enough to fit all the ramekins, add 1 inch of water. Cover the pan and heat the water on medium heat until it reaches a simmer.
5. Carefully place the ramekins in the water bath, cover, and cook on medium heat for 3 minutes.

Note: You will need six 1-cup ramekins for this recipe.
Note: Instead of salmon, you may use ham, shrimp, or any other cooked lean protein.

Curried Hard-Boiled Eggs

MAKES 1 SERVING
Preparation time: 10 minutes
Cooking time: 25 minutes

2 eggs
½ cup fat-free milk
1 tablespoon finely chopped onion
A pinch of cornstarch (see Note)
Salt and freshly ground black pepper
1 teaspoon curry powder

1. Place eggs in a small pot and cover with cold water. Bring to a boil. Once the water is boiling, reduce heat to a simmer and cook the eggs for 10 minutes.
2. While eggs are cooking, add ¼ cup of the milk and the chopped onion to a small saucepan and cook over medium heat for 10 minutes, stirring continuously.
3. In a small bowl whisk together the cornstarch and the remaining cold milk.
4. Add the milk and cornstarch mixture, salt and pepper to taste, and the curry powder to the warm milk and onion, and mix until thoroughly incorporated.
5. Remove the eggs from the pot and help them to cool by running cold water over them. Peel and slice the eggs and arrange on a serving dish. Pour the sauce over the eggs, and serve warm.

Note: You may eat this dish only on pure protein days during the Cruise phase, not during the Attack phase.

Tuna Omelet

MAKES 4 SERVINGS
Preparation time: 10 minutes
Cooking time: 5 minutes

8 eggs
2 anchovy fillets, minced
1 (5-ounce) can of tuna packed in water, drained, and flaked
1 tablespoon chopped fresh parsley
Freshly ground black pepper
⅛ teaspoon vegetable oil

1. In a medium bowl, beat the eggs, add the anchovy and tuna, and mix until combined.
2. Season with the parsley and pepper to taste.
3. Heat a medium nonstick skillet over medium heat. Add the oil and wipe out any excess with a paper towel.
4. Add the egg mixture to the skillet and cook to your liking. Serve immediately.

Eggs Stuffed with Tuna

MAKES 4 SERVINGS
Preparation time: 15 minutes
Cooking time: 20 minutes

4 eggs
1 (5-ounce) can of tuna packed in water, well drained
1 tablespoon fat-free plain Greek-style yogurt
1 tablespoon fat-free ricotta
1 teaspoon mustard
Salt and freshly ground black pepper

1. Place eggs in a large pot and cover with cold water. Bring to a boil. Once the water is boiling, reduce heat to a simmer and

cook the eggs for 10 minutes. Remove the eggs from the hot water and help them cool by running cold water over them.

2. Peel the eggs and cut them in half lengthways.
3. Place the yolks in a medium bowl and reserve the whites.
4. Add the tuna, yogurt, ricotta, and mustard to the egg yolks, along with salt and pepper to taste.
5. Using a fork, mash the yolks with the other ingredients until you have a paste.
6. Divide the mixture evenly among the egg white halves, then place 2 halves together to make them into "whole eggs" again.
7. Place in the refrigerator until ready to eat.

Crab Flan

MAKES 5 SERVINGS
Preparation time: 10 minutes
Cooking time: 30 minutes

⅛ teaspoon vegetable oil
7 ounces smoked salmon, diced
1 tablespoon cornstarch
¾ cup fat-free milk
2 eggs
1 (6-ounce) can of white crabmeat, well drained
Salt and freshly ground black pepper
¼ teaspoon low-sodium fish stock

1. Preheat oven to 350°F.
2. Divide the oil evenly among five 1-cup ramekins and wipe out excess with a paper towel.
3. Divide the smoked salmon among the ramekins.
4. In a small bowl, combine the cornstarch and milk, and beat until smooth.
5. Add the eggs, mix until smooth, and then add the crabmeat.
6. Season with salt and pepper to taste and add the fish stock.

7. Divide the mixture among the ramekins. Place the ramekins into a bigger baking dish large enough to fit them. Fill the bigger baking dish halfway with cold water. Bake for 30 minutes.

Note: You will need five 1-cup ramekins for this recipe.

Crustless Chicken Quiche

MAKES 2 SERVINGS
Preparation time: 15 minutes
Cooking time: 20 minutes

⅛ teaspoon vegetable oil
6 tablespoons fat-free ricotta
3 eggs, beaten
2 slices of cooked skinless chicken, cut into small pieces
½ onion, chopped
A pinch of ground nutmeg
Salt and freshly ground black pepper

1. Preheat oven to 475°F.
2. Add the oil to a 4-cup baking dish, using a paper towel to coat it and to wipe out any excess.
3. In a medium bowl, mix together the ricotta, eggs, chicken, onion, and nutmeg, along with salt and pepper to taste.
4. Pour the egg mixture into the baking dish and bake for 20 minutes.

Ham Soufflé

MAKES 4 SERVINGS
Preparation time: 15 minutes
Cooking time: 45 minutes

⅛ teaspoon vegetable oil
½ cup fat-free milk
¾ teaspoon cornstarch (see Note)
4 eggs, separated
1¾ cups fat-free plain Greek-style yogurt
7 ounces extra-lean ham, cut into strips
A pinch of ground nutmeg
Salt and freshly ground black pepper

1. Preheat oven to 425°F.
2. Add the oil to an 8-inch nonstick soufflé dish, using a paper towel to wipe out any excess.
3. In a large bowl, combine milk and cornstarch and mix until smooth.
4. In a medium bowl, beat the egg yolks with the yogurt then pour over the milk, stirring constantly to obtain a smooth paste.
5. Add the ham and nutmeg and season with salt and pepper to taste.
6. In a medium mixing bowl, beat the egg whites until very stiff.
7. Carefully fold the egg whites into the ham mixture.
8. Pour the mixture into the prepared soufflé dish.
9. Bake in the oven for 45 minutes. Serve immediately.

Note: You will need an 8-inch nonstick soufflé dish for this recipe.
Note: You may eat this dish only on pure protein days during the Cruise phase, not during the Attack phase.

Salmon and Egg Terrine

MAKES 8 TO 10 SERVINGS

Preparation time: 30 minutes, plus overnight refrigeration

Cooking time: 20 minutes

10 eggs

½ cup chopped mixed fresh herbs, such as parsley, chives, and tarragon

4 ounces sliced smoked salmon

2 (7-gram) envelopes of unflavored gelatin

½ cup Dukan Mayonnaise (page 331)

1. Place eggs in a large pot and cover with cold water. Bring to a boil. Once the water is boiling, reduce heat to a simmer and cook the eggs for 10 minutes.
2. Remove the eggs from the hot water and help them cool by running cold water over them.
3. Remove shells and chop.
4. In a small bowl mix the eggs with half the herbs.
5. Place a third of the egg mixture in the bottom of an 8 × 4-inch loaf pan and then top with a third of the salmon. Repeat two more times, using all of the eggs and salmon.
6. In a medium bowl, combine the gelatin with ¼ cup cold water and let stand for 1 minute.
7. Add 1 cup hot water to the gelatin mixture and stir until dissolved.
8. Pour the gelatin mixture over the terrine.
9. Cover and refrigerate overnight.
10. Before serving, add the remaining herbs to the mayonnaise.
11. To turn the terrine out of the pan, immerse the bottom of the pan in some hot water then invert it onto a large plate. The terrine will slide out. Serve the terrine cut into slices with the herb mayonnaise on the side.

Note: You will need an 8 × 4-inch loaf pan for this recipe. Prepare the terrine the day before you wish to eat it.

Shirataki Noodles

Shirataki noodles were developed in Asia. Made of yam starch, they are very high in fiber and very low in carbohydrates and calories, making them an ideal food for the Dukan dieter. They can be added to soups or stir-fries, integrated into any protein dish, or simply prepared like pasta and served with your favorite sauce.

The noodles need to be drained from their packaging, rinsed, and cooked before you use them in a recipe. The noodles can be bought from our website: www.shopdukandiet.com.

To prepare shirataki noodles on the stovetop:

1. Remove the noodles from their packaging, drain in a colander, and rinse thoroughly under cold running water.
2. Fill a medium saucepan with water and bring to a boil.
3. Add the noodles, return the water to a boil, and cook for 2 minutes.
4. Drain the noodles, rinse again, and pat dry with a paper towel. Use as desired.

To prepare shirataki noodles in the microwave:

1. Remove the noodles from their packaging, drain in a colander, and rinse thoroughly under cold running water.
2. Place the noodles in a microwave-safe dish and cook for 1 minute.
3. Drain the noodles, rinse again, and pat dry with a paper towel. Use as desired.

Chicken Tandoori and Shirataki Noodles

MAKES 1 SERVING

Preparation time: 10 minutes, plus 30 minutes for marinating

Cooking time: 5 minutes

½ cup fat-free plain Greek-style yogurt

¼ teaspoon garam masala

¼ teaspoon curry powder

Salt and freshly ground black pepper

1 boneless, skinless chicken breast, cut into strips

1 (7-ounce) package of shirataki noodles, such as Dukan Diet
   Shirataki Noodles, prepared according to the directions on
   page 87.

1. In a small bowl, combine the yogurt, garam masala, and curry powder, along with salt and pepper to taste.
2. Place the chicken in a shallow bowl and coat with the yogurt mixture.
3. Cover the chicken, refrigerate, and let marinate for at least 30 minutes.
4. Preheat oven to Broil for 5 minutes.
5. Transfer the chicken to a baking sheet, broil for 2 minutes, then remove the pan from the broiler and stir the mixture. Return the pan to the oven and continue broiling until the chicken is cooked through, about 3 additional minutes.
6. In a large bowl, toss cooked noodles and chicken together until thoroughly combined. Serve warm or at room temperature.

Turkey with Shirataki Noodles

MAKES 4 SERVINGS

Preparation time: 10 minutes

Cooking time: 15 minutes

1 pound lean ground turkey breast

2 tablespoons ground cumin

1 tablespoon ground coriander seeds

1 tablespoon fennel seeds

Freshly ground black pepper

3 (7-ounce) packages of shirataki noodles, such as Dukan Diet
Shirataki Noodles, prepared according to the directions on
page 87.

1 scallion, white and green parts, finely sliced (optional)

1. Heat a large nonstick pan over medium heat.
2. Add the ground turkey, cumin, coriander, and fennel, along
   with pepper to taste.
3. Cook, stirring often, until browned, about 10 minutes.
4. Add the noodles and scallion to the turkey mixture and cook
   for another 5 minutes.
5. Serve hot.

Note: During the Cruise phase, add shredded or chopped vegetables,
such as cabbage, carrots, and mushrooms.

Indian-Style Chicken with Shirataki Noodles

MAKES 4 SERVINGS

Preparation time: 10 minutes, plus overnight marinating

Cooking time: 10 minutes

1½ cups fat-free plain Greek-style yogurt

2 tablespoons tandoori spice mix, or 1 teaspoon each of ground ginger, ground cumin, ground coriander, paprika, turmeric, and salt, plus cayenne pepper

4 boneless, skinless chicken breasts, cut into ¼-inch strips

⅛ teaspoon vegetable oil

3 (7-ounce) packages of shirataki noodles, such as Dukan Diet Shirataki Noodles, prepared according to the directions on page 87.

Salt and freshly ground black pepper

1. In a shallow bowl, combine the yogurt and tandoori spice mix. Add the chicken strips, toss thoroughly, cover, and refrigerate overnight.

2. The next day, when ready to cook, drain the chicken, reserving the marinade.

3. Heat a large nonstick pan over medium heat. Add the oil and wipe out any excess with a paper towel.

4. Add the chicken and cook, stirring often, for 5 minutes.

5. Add the cooked noodles and reserved marinade and cook, stirring often, until thoroughly heated, about 5 minutes. Season with salt and pepper to taste.

Note: This recipe, including the noodles, is delicious served over steamed green beans in the Cruise phase.

Discover Dukan Diet Shirataki Noodles

Seafood and Fish

Shrimp Frittata

MAKES 2 SERVINGS

Preparation time: 10 minutes

Cooking time: 30 minutes

4 eggs

Salt and freshly ground black pepper

1 cup fat-free plain Greek-style yogurt

10 ounces shelled shrimp, coarsely chopped

⅛ teaspoon vegetable oil

1. Preheat oven to 400°F.
2. In a medium bowl, beat the eggs and season with salt and pepper to taste. Gradually add the yogurt, stirring thoroughly.
3. Add the shrimp to the egg mixture.
4. Add the oil to a 4-cup baking dish, using a paper towel to coat it and to wipe out any excess.
5. Place shrimp/egg mixture in the baking dish and bake for 30 minutes.

Potted Shrimp

MAKES 2 SERVINGS

Preparation time: 10 minutes

Cooking time: No cooking required

1 tablespoon very finely chopped fresh dill

6 tablespoons Dukan Mayonnaise (page 331)

10 ounces cooked shelled shrimp, roughly chopped

2 pinches of paprika

Freshly ground black pepper

1. In a medium bowl, combine the dill and the mayonnaise.
2. Add the shrimp, mix in the paprika, and add pepper to taste.

Scallop Mousse

MAKES 4 SERVINGS
Preparation time: 15 minutes
Cooking time: 10 minutes

8 sea scallops, cut in half across the grain, or 24 whole bay
 scallops
1 cup fat-free plain Greek-style yogurt
2 eggs, separated
Salt and freshly ground black pepper
⅛ teaspoon vegetable oil
Lemon and Chive Sauce (see page 340)

1. In a large bowl, mix the scallops with the yogurt. Add the egg yolks and salt and pepper to taste.
2. In a mixing bowl, beat the egg whites until stiff.
3. Gently fold the egg whites into the scallop mixture.
4. Distribute the oil among four 1-cup ramekins, using a paper towel to coat them and to wipe out any excess.
5. Divide the egg and scallop mixture among the ramekins.
6. Fill the bottom part of a large steamer with water and bring to a simmer.
7. Place the ramekins in the top part of the steamer, cover, and steam for 10 minutes.
8. Serve the mousse hot with Lemon and Chive Sauce.

Note: You will need a large steamer and four 1-cup ramekins for this recipe.

Seafood Omelet

MAKES 3 SERVINGS
Preparation time: 20 minutes
Cooking time: 20 minutes

⅛ teaspoon vegetable oil
2 eggs
1 cup fat-free milk
1 (6-ounce) can of white crabmeat, drained
5 ounces cooked, shelled shrimp
5 ounces cooked, shelled mussels
Salt and freshly ground black pepper

1. Preheat oven to 425°F.
2. Distribute the oil among three 1-cup ramekins, using a paper towel to coat the ramekins, and wiping out any excess.
3. In a medium bowl, beat the eggs and milk until thoroughly combined.
4. Add the crabmeat, shrimp, and mussels to the egg mixture, along with salt and pepper to taste. Mix thoroughly.
5. Divide the mixture among the prepared ramekins.
6. Place the ramekins into a baking dish large enough to fit them, and fill the baking dish half full with cold water.
7. Place the baking dish in the oven and bake the omelets for 20 minutes or until set. Serve hot.

Note: You will need three 1-cup ramekins for this recipe.

Tilapia with Aromatic Herbs

MAKES 2 SERVINGS

Preparation time: 25 minutes

Cooking time: 5 minutes

¼ cup white wine vinegar

12 ounces tilapia fillets

1 large bunch of fresh herbs, such as chives, parsley, and
tarragon

Salt and freshly ground black pepper

Juice ½ a lemon

1 tablespoon finely chopped mixed fresh herbs, such as chives,
parsley, and tarragon

1. Fill the bottom portion of a large steamer with water, bring
   to a simmer, and add the vinegar to the water.
2. Cover the top portion of the steamer with the whole herbs
   and place the tilapia on top.
3. Add salt and pepper to taste, cover, and steam for 5 minutes.
4. Remove the fish from the steamer and sprinkle with the
   lemon juice.
5. Serve the fish garnished with the chopped herbs.

Note: You will need a large steamer for this recipe.

Tilapia in a Creamy Tarragon Sauce

MAKES 2 SERVINGS

Preparation time: 20 minutes

Cooking time: 20 minutes

12 ounces tilapia fillets

1 teaspoon white wine vinegar

3 bay leaves

2 tablespoons tarragon vinegar

1 shallot, chopped

Salt and freshly ground black pepper

1 tablespoon capers, drained and rinsed

½ cup fat-free plain Greek-style yogurt

1 tablespoon chopped fresh parsley

1. Place the tilapia in a saucepan just large enough to hold the fish.
2. Add the white wine vinegar, bay leaves, and enough water to just barely cover the fish.
3. Bring the liquid to a simmer and cook until fish is opaque in the center, about 5 minutes.
4. In the meantime, add the shallot and tarragon vinegar to a saucepan, along with salt and pepper to taste. Cook over medium heat until the shallot begins to brown and most of the liquid is evaporated.
5. Turn the heat to low, add the capers and yogurt, and cook, stirring constantly, until heated through. Do not allow the sauce to boil.
6. Remove the fish from the poaching liquid with a slotted spoon. Serve it covered with the yogurt sauce and garnished with the chopped parsley.

Cod with Mustard Sauce

MAKES 1 SERVING
Preparation time: 10 minutes
Cooking time: 15 minutes

⅛ teaspoon vegetable oil

7-ounce cod fillet

Salt and freshly ground black pepper

¾ cup fat-free plain Greek-style yogurt

1 tablespoon mustard

1 teaspoon fresh lemon juice

2 tablespoons capers, drained and rinsed

1 bunch of fresh parsley, leaves finely chopped and stems
    discarded

1. Fill the bottom part of a large steamer with water and bring to a simmer.

2. Coat the top part of the steamer with the oil and use a paper towel to wipe out any excess. Add the cod and season with salt and pepper to taste.

3. Cover the steamer and cook the fish until it is opaque in the center, about 5 minutes for a ½-inch-thick fillet, 10 minutes for a 1-inch-thick fillet.

4. In the meantime, put the yogurt, mustard, lemon juice, capers, and parsley into a saucepan, along with pepper to taste.

5. Heat the yogurt mixture over low heat, stirring constantly. Do not let the sauce boil.

6. Place the cooked fish on a serving dish, pour the sauce over the fish, and serve.

Note: You will need a large steamer for this recipe.

Cod with Shallots and Mustard

MAKES 2 SERVINGS
Preparation time: 15 minutes
Cooking time: 15 minutes

4 shallots, chopped
¼ cup fat-free plain Greek-style yogurt
1 tablespoon mustard
2 tablespoons lemon juice
Salt and freshly ground black pepper
14-ounce cod fillet, divided into 2 portions

1. Preheat oven to 350°F.
2. Place shallots in a saucepan with 1 tablespoon water and cook over medium heat until the shallots turn translucent.
3. In a small bowl, mix together the yogurt, mustard, and lemon juice, along with salt and pepper to taste.
4. Cover the bottom of a 9-inch glass pie plate with the cooked shallots.
5. Place the cod on top of the shallots and pour the yogurt sauce over the fish.
6. Place the dish in the oven and bake the fish until it is opaque in the center, about 10 minutes.

Spicy Indian Cod

MAKES 2 SERVINGS
Preparation time: 20 minutes
Cooking time: 20 minutes

14-ounce cod fillet, divided into 2 portions
1½ cups low-sodium vegetable stock
⅛ teaspoon vegetable oil
1 medium onion, chopped
1 egg yolk
½ teaspoon curry powder
A pinch of saffron
Salt and freshly ground black pepper
1 tablespoon chopped fresh parsley

1. Place the cod in a saucepan just large enough to hold the fish.
2. Add 1 cup of the vegetable stock, bring to a simmer, and cook the fish until it is opaque in the center, about 5 minutes for a ½-inch-thick fillet, 10 minutes for a 1-inch-thick fillet.
3. In the meantime, heat a large nonstick frying pan over medium heat.
4. Add the oil and wipe out any excess with a paper towel.
5. Add the onion and cook until brown, about 5 minutes.
6. Add the remaining ½ cup of the vegetable stock and reduce for 2 minutes.
7. Add the egg yolk, diluted in a little of the hot liquid, stirring constantly. Continuing to stir, allow the sauce to gradually thicken.
8. Season the sauce with curry powder and saffron, and add salt and pepper to taste. Continue cooking, without allowing the sauce to boil, for an additional 5 minutes.
9. Arrange the fish fillets in a hot serving dish, pour the sauce over them, and garnish with the parsley.

Cod with Creamy Caper Sauce

MAKES 2 SERVINGS
Preparation time: 15 minutes
Cooking time: 10 minutes

14-ounce cod fillet, divided into 2 portions
1 bay leaf
3 peppercorns
Salt
¾ cup fat-free plain Greek-style yogurt
1 egg yolk
2 tablespoons fresh lemon juice
2 tablespoons capers, drained and rinsed
1 tablespoon finely chopped fresh flat-leaf parsley
1 tablespoon finely chopped fresh chives

1. Place the cod in a large nonstick, high-sided frying pan with the bay leaf, peppercorns, and salt to taste.
2. Cover the cod with cold water, bring to a simmer over low heat, and cook the fish until it is opaque in the center, about 5 minutes for a ½-inch-thick fillet, 10 minutes for a 1-inch-thick fillet.
3. While fish is cooking, pour the yogurt into a small saucepan and heat gently.
4. In a medium bowl, mix together the egg yolk and lemon juice, then add to the yogurt, stirring vigorously until the sauce starts to simmer.
5. Add the capers, parsley, and chives.
6. Remove the fish from the poaching liquid with a slotted spoon, place it on a serving dish, and pour the sauce over it.

Trout Terrine

MAKES 3 TO 4 SERVINGS
Preparation time: 20 minutes
Cooking time: 25 minutes

1¼ pounds skinless trout fillets

7 cups low-sodium vegetable stock

1 egg

2 tablespoons fat-free plain Greek-style yogurt

1 tablespoon finely chopped fresh herbs, such as basil, tarragon, or cilantro

Salt and freshly ground black pepper

⅛ teaspoon vegetable oil

1. Preheat oven to 350°F.
2. Place the trout in a large saucepan.
3. Add the vegetable stock, bring to a simmer, and cook until the fish is opaque in the center, about 5 minutes.
4. Remove the trout from the poaching liquid and purée in a blender.
5. Add the egg, yogurt, and herbs, along with salt and pepper to taste, and process until smooth.
6. Distribute the oil among three or four 1-cup ramekins, using a paper towel to coat the ramekins, and wiping out any excess.
7. Divide the fish mixture among the prepared ramekins.
8. Place the ramekins in a larger baking dish, and fill the larger baking dish halfway with cold water.
9. Place the baking dish in the oven, and bake the terrine for 20 minutes or until set.

Note: You will need three or four 1-cup ramekins for this recipe.

Salmon Cutlets in a Mustard Dill Sauce

MAKES 4 SERVINGS

Preparation time: 20 minutes

Cooking time: 15 minutes

1¾ pounds skinless salmon fillets, divided into 4 portions

2 shallots, chopped

1 tablespoon mild mustard

2 tablespoons fat-free plain Greek-style yogurt

2 tablespoons finely chopped fresh dill

Salt and freshly ground black pepper

1. Put the salmon in the freezer for a few minutes, remove, and cut into ½-inch-thick slices.
2. Heat a large nonstick frying pan over medium heat, and cook the salmon for 30 seconds on each side for medium-rare, 1 minute on each side for more well done. Depending on the size of your pan, you may need to cook the salmon in more than one batch.
3. Once the salmon is cooked, remove it from the pan and keep it warm.
4. Brown the shallots in the same frying pan.
5. Once the shallots are browned, reduce the heat to low and add the mustard and yogurt.
6. Cook this mixture slowly, stirring often, until thick, about 5 minutes.
7. Return the salmon to the frying pan with the sauce. Add the dill, along with salt and pepper to taste.
8. Heat thoroughly and serve immediately.

Pink and White Frittata

MAKES 3 SERVINGS

Preparation time: 10 minutes

Cooking time: 20 minutes

1 tablespoon cornstarch (see Note)

1 pound flounder fillets, chopped into small pieces

3 eggs, beaten

½ cup fat-free plain Greek-style yogurt

Salt and freshly ground black pepper

⅛ teaspoon vegetable oil

5 ounces skinless salmon fillet

1. Preheat oven to 425°F.
2. In a medium bowl, combine the cornstarch with 1 tablespoon cold water.
3. Mix in the flounder, eggs, and yogurt, along with salt and pepper to taste.
4. Add the oil to a 9-inch loaf pan, using a paper towel to coat it and to wipe out any excess.
5. Pour the flounder mixture into the loaf pan, and place the salmon fillet in the middle of the mixture.
6. Bake in the oven for 20 minutes.

Note: You will need a 9-inch loaf pan for this recipe.

Note: You may eat this dish only on pure protein days during the Cruise phase, not during the Attack phase.

Smoked Salmon Roll

MAKES 3 SERVINGS

Preparation time: 10 minutes, plus 3 hours for refrigeration

Cooking time: 15 minutes

3 eggs

1 tablespoon cornstarch (see Note)

⅛ teaspoon vegetable oil

1 cup fat-free ricotta

2 tablespoons chopped fresh chives

1 tablespoon peeled and chopped fresh ginger

3½ ounces smoked salmon, chopped

Freshly ground black pepper

A few sprigs of fresh parsley

1. In a small bowl, mix together 1 egg, 1 tablespoon water, and 1 teaspoon of the cornstarch.
2. Heat a large nonstick frying pan over medium heat. Add the oil and wipe out any excess with a paper towel.
3. Pour the egg mixture into the frying pan and make a thin omelet. Do not fold; it should look like a thin pancake, or crêpe.
5. Place the cooked omelet on a plate and repeat the process to make two more omelets, using another ⅛ teaspoon oil, if necessary.
6. Divide the ricotta evenly into three portions and carefully spread over each omelet.
7. Top each omelet with chives, ginger, salmon, and pepper to taste.
8. Roll each omelet tightly, wrap in plastic wrap, and refrigerate for 3 hours.
9. Using a very sharp knife, cut each omelet roll into slices. Serve garnished with parsley.

Note: You may eat this dish only on pure protein days during the Cruise phase, not during the Attack phase.

Herb-Stuffed Baked Salmon

MAKES 6 SERVINGS

Preparation time: 20 minutes, plus 2 to 3 hours for marinating

Cooking time: 25 minutes

1 bunch of fresh flat-leaf parsley, chopped

1 bunch of fresh cilantro, chopped

½ cup chopped fresh mild green chilies

5 fresh lemongrass stalks, chopped

1 cup chopped shallots

4 garlic cloves, chopped

1 lemon, cut into very thin slices

1 teaspoon ground cumin

1 teaspoon peeled and grated fresh ginger

½ cup white wine

Salt and freshly ground black pepper

1 whole salmon, approximately 3½ pounds, cleaned, scaled, and with central bone removed (this can be done at your local grocery's fish counter)

1. In a medium bowl, combine the parsley, cilantro, chilies, lemongrass, shallots, garlic, lemon slices, cumin, ginger, and white wine, plus salt and pepper to taste.
2. Place the salmon on a tray and coat both sides of the fish with the marinade.
3. Wrap the salmon and place it in the refrigerator for 2 to 3 hours to marinate.
4. Preheat oven to 400°F.
5. Open up the salmon, season it with salt and pepper to taste, and fill it with the marinade.
6. Place the salmon on a baking pan lined with a sheet of non-stick foil or parchment paper, and bake for 25 minutes.

Salmon and Monkfish Terrine with Lime

MAKES 3 TO 4 SERVINGS

Preparation time: 30 minutes, plus 1 hour for marinating and
4 hours for refrigeration

Cooking time: No cooking required

14 ounces skinless salmon fillet, cut into ⅛-inch-thick slices

7 ounces skinless monkfish fillet, cut into ⅛-inch-thick slices

⅓ cup fresh lime juice

1 drop of Tabasco sauce

A pinch of ground nutmeg

Freshly ground black pepper

2 (7-gram) envelopes of unflavored gelatin

1 teaspoon crushed pink peppercorns

4 small white onions, chopped

2 tablespoons finely chopped fresh basil

1. Place salmon and monkfish in a shallow dish.
2. In a medium bowl, mix together the lime juice, Tabasco, and nutmeg, along with pepper to taste.
3. Pour lime marinade over the fish, cover, and marinate for 1 hour in the refrigerator.
4. While the fish is marinating, place the gelatin in a medium bowl and mix with ¼ cup cold water. Let stand for 1 minute.
5. Add 2 cups hot water to the gelatin and stir until thoroughly dissolved.
6. Allow the gelatin to cool to room temperature.
7. Drain the fish; discard the marinade.
8. Line a deep 9-inch loaf pan with plastic wrap (the pan should be able to hold at least 4 cups of liquid). Make sure the plastic wrap overlaps the edges generously.
9. Pour a thin layer of the gelatin into the bottom of the pan and place in refrigerator until it is set, about 5 minutes.
10. Top the gelatin with alternating layers of salmon and monkfish, starting and ending with salmon. In between each layer scatter crushed peppercorns, onions, and basil.

11. Pour the remaining gelatin over the fish.
12. Shake the pan a little so that the gelatin fills any gaps.
13. Fold the plastic wrap over the top to completely cover the pan and place it in the refrigerator to set for at least 4 hours.
14. To serve, remove the terrine from the loaf pan, discard the plastic wrap, and slice.

Note: You will need a 9-inch loaf pan for this recipe.
Note: Eating raw fish carries some risk of food-borne illness. Raw fish should not be consumed by the very young, the very old, pregnant women, or anyone with a compromised immune system.

Smoked Salmon Appetizers

MAKES 2 SERVINGS
Preparation time: 5 minutes
Cooking time: No cooking required

1¼ cups fat-free ricotta
¼ cup fat-free plain Greek-style yogurt
1 (2-ounce) jar of salmon roe
Salt and freshly ground black pepper
4 slices of smoked salmon
4 long chives or wooden toothpicks

1. In a medium bowl, combine the ricotta and yogurt.
2. Carefully fold in the salmon roe and season with salt and pepper to taste.
3. Divide the ricotta mixture among the salmon slices.
4. Roll up each slice of salmon and keep it in place by tying it with a chive or by piercing it with a toothpick.
5. Cover and keep refrigerated until ready to serve.

Note: Serve with some mini Dukan Oat Bran Galettes (page 120).

Spicy Red Snapper Tartare

MAKES 6 SERVINGS

Preparation time: 15 minutes

Cooking time: No cooking required

2½ pounds red snapper fillets

1 cucumber

¼ cup fresh lemon juice

3 shallots, chopped

1 bunch of fresh herbs, such as flat-leaf parsley, dill, chervil,
    or chives, chopped

A few drops of Tabasco sauce

Salt and freshly ground black pepper

1. Roughly chop the fish in a food processor by pulsing on and off.
2. Peel the cucumber and cut into small pieces.
3. In a large bowl, mix the fish, cucumber, lemon juice, shallots, and herbs.
4. Season with the Tabasco, and add salt and pepper to taste.
5. Cover and refrigerate until ready to serve.

Note: Eating raw fish carries some risk of food-borne illness. Raw fish should not be consumed by the very young, the very old, pregnant women, or anyone with a compromised immune system.

Red Snapper with Saffron

MAKES 1 SERVING

Preparation time: 15 minutes

Cooking time: 10 minutes

⅛ teaspoon vegetable oil

5½ ounces red snapper fillet

Salt and freshly ground black pepper

A pinch of saffron

¾ cup fat-free plain Greek-style yogurt

1. Preheat oven to 425°F.
2. Add the oil to a medium baking dish, using a paper towel to coat it and to wipe out any excess.
3. Place the snapper in the baking dish and season with salt and pepper to taste.
4. In a small bowl, mix the saffron into the yogurt and spread over the fish.
5. Cover the baking dish with a sheet of aluminum foil and bake the fish until it is opaque in the center, about 10 minutes.

Salt-Crusted Red Snapper

MAKES 4 SERVINGS

Preparation time: 10 minutes

Cooking time: 50 minutes

1 whole red snapper, weighing 2¼ to 3¼ pounds, cleaned but with skin and scales left on

2 cups coarse sea salt

1. Preheat oven to 450°F.
2. Select a casserole slightly larger than the fish. Line the inside with aluminum foil.
3. Fill the bottom of the casserole with a layer of salt 1 inch thick.

4. Place the fish on top of the salt and cover it with the remaining salt. The fish should be completely covered with the salt.
5. Sprinkle the top with a little water to form the crust.
6. Place the casserole in the oven and bake the fish for 30 minutes. Then lower the temperature to 350°F and continue cooking for 20 minutes more.
7. Turn the contents of the casserole out onto a cutting board, and break the salt crust with the back of a spoon or a hammer.
8. Brush away the salt and carefully remove the skin from the fish before serving.

Baked Red Snapper with Onion Compote

MAKES 2 SERVINGS
Preparation time: 15 minutes
Cooking time: 10 minutes

⅛ teaspoon vegetable oil
1 large onion, chopped
10 ounces red snapper fillets, divided into 2 portions
Salt and freshly ground black pepper
1 tablespoon fresh parsley, chopped

1. Preheat oven to 350°F.
2. Heat a large nonstick skillet over low heat, add the oil, and wipe out any excess with a paper towel.
3. Add the onion and cook, stirring constantly, until the onion is soft but not browned.
4. Cut two sheets of foil or parchment paper, each twice the size of the fish portion, and divide the onion between the two.
5. Place each fish portion on its bed of onion, then season with salt and pepper to taste.
6. Wrap up each portion in the foil, seal it, and place it in a baking dish.

7. Cook the two parcels until the fish is opaque in the middle, about 10 minutes.
8. Take care when opening the parcels because they will be very hot. Garnish the fish with the parsley.

Baked Fish with Herbs

MAKES 4 SERVINGS
Preparation time: 15 minutes
Cooking time: 30 minutes

1¾ pounds fish fillets, such as red snapper or cod
Salt and freshly ground black pepper
1¼ cups fat-free plain Greek-style yogurt
4 eggs
5 tablespoons chopped fresh herbs of your choice, such as
    parsley, tarragon, and chives
⅛ teaspoon vegetable oil

1. Preheat oven to 425°F. Line a baking sheet with foil or parchment paper.
2. Arrange fillets on baking sheet and season with salt and pepper to taste.
3. Bake the fish until it is opaque in the center, about 5 minutes.
4. Remove the fish from the oven and reduce the oven temperature to 350°F.
5. Put the fish, yogurt, eggs, and herbs into a blender and process until smooth, about 45 seconds.
6. Add the oil to a 6-cup baking dish, using a paper towel to coat it and to wipe out any excess.
7. Fill the prepared baking dish with the fish mixture and place it into a larger ovenproof dish.
8. Fill the larger dish half full with cold water and bake the fish mixture until it is set, about 25 minutes.

Sea Bass Tartare

MAKES 2 SERVINGS
Preparation time: 20 minutes
Cooking time: No cooking required

14 ounces sea bass fillet
2 shallots, finely chopped
½ cup fat-free plain Greek-style yogurt
1 tablespoon fresh lemon juice
Salt and freshly ground black pepper
A few fresh chives, finely chopped

1. With a knife, cut the fish up roughly into very small pieces, place in a large bowl, and mix with the shallots.
2. In a small bowl, combine the yogurt and lemon juice, and season with salt and pepper to taste.
3. To serve, top the fish with the yogurt sauce and garnish with the chives. Serve immediately, or cover and refrigerate until ready to serve.

Note: Eating raw fish carries some risk of food-borne illness. Raw fish should not be consumed by the very young, the very old, pregnant women, or anyone with a compromised immune system.
Note: During the Cruise phase, you may serve this recipe with 4 lime wedges (2 per serving) or on a bed of lettuce.

Mint and Cinnamon–Scented Sea Bass

MAKES 4 SERVINGS

Preparation time: 10 minutes

Cooking time: 5 minutes

½ teaspoon ground cinnamon

3 sprigs of fresh mint

⅛ teaspoon vegetable oil

1¼ pounds sea bass fillets, skin on, divided into 4 pieces

Salt and freshly ground black pepper

½ lemon

2 cinnamon sticks, each cut in half

1. Fill the bottom of a large steamer with water and add the ground cinnamon and 2 of the mint sprigs. Bring the water to a simmer.
2. Coat the top part of the steamer with the oil and use a paper towel to wipe out any excess.
3. Add the fish, season with salt and pepper to taste, cover, and cook until the fillets are opaque in the center, about 5 minutes.
4. Squeeze the half lemon over the fish before serving and garnish with mint leaves from the reserved sprig, plus half a cinnamon stick for each portion.

Note: You will need a large steamer for this recipe.

Breton-Style Bluefish

MAKES 3 SERVINGS

Preparation time: 15 minutes

Cooking time: 20 minutes

1¼ pounds bluefish fillets, divided into 3 pieces

3 shallots, chopped

1 small bunch of fresh parsley, chopped

2 tablespoons chopped fresh chives

3 tablespoons cider vinegar

1. Preheat oven to 400°F.
2. Place each portion of the fish on a piece of aluminum foil or parchment paper twice the size of the fish portion.
3. Top each piece of fish with the shallots, parsley, and chives and 1 tablespoon of the vinegar.
4. Seal the fish carefully inside the aluminum foil and place on a baking sheet. Place in the oven, and bake for 20 minutes.
5. Take care when opening the fish packets, because they will be very hot.

Bluefish Rillettes

MAKES 4 SERVINGS
Preparation time: 20 minutes
Cooking time: 20 minutes

2¼ pounds skinless bluefish fillets
8½ cups cold low-sodium fish stock
1 teaspoon coarse sea salt
5 tablespoons tarragon- or green peppercorn–flavored mustard
2 tablespoons fresh lemon juice
3 tablespoons finely chopped fresh parsley or chives
⅛ teaspoon vegetable oil

1. Place the fish in a large pot and add the cold fish stock and salt.
2. Warm over high heat and as soon as the liquid starts to boil, turn off the heat, cover the pot, and let it sit for 2 minutes.
3. Remove the fish to a plate and let it cool.
4. Place the fish in a large bowl and mash it with a fork.
5. In a small bowl, combine the mustard, lemon juice, and 2 tablespoons of the parsley or chives.
6. Add the mustard mixture to the fish and combine thoroughly.
7. Distribute the oil among four 2-cup ramekins, using a paper towel to coat them and to wipe out any excess.

8. Press the fish mixture into the containers and decorate them with the remaining tablespoon of parsley or chives.

Note: You will need four 2-cup ramekins for this recipe. During the Cruise phase, you may serve this recipe with ½ lemon, cut in wedges.

Tuna Tartare

MAKES 4 SERVINGS

Preparation time: 15 minutes, plus 15 minutes for marinating

Cooking time: No cooking required

2¼ pounds Ahi tuna steaks
3 tablespoons fresh lime juice
1 garlic clove, crushed
1 tablespoon peeled and grated fresh ginger
2 tablespoons finely chopped fresh chives
1 tablespoon fat-free plain Greek-style yogurt
Salt and freshly ground black pepper

1. Cut the tuna up into ½-inch cubes, place in a large bowl, and toss with the lime juice.
2. In a medium bowl, combine the garlic, ginger, chives, and yogurt. Season with salt and pepper to taste.
3. Add the dressing to the fish and mix thoroughly.
4. Cover and refrigerate for 15 minutes before serving.

Note: Eating raw fish carries some risk of food-borne illness. Raw fish should not be consumed by the very young, the very old, pregnant women, or anyone with a compromised immune system.

Tuna and Red Snapper Tartare

MAKES 6 SERVINGS

Preparation time: 20 minutes, plus 15 minutes for marinating

Cooking time: No cooking required

14 ounces Ahi tuna steaks

14 ounces skinless red snapper fillets

1 tablespoon tarragon vinegar

3 tablespoons fresh lime juice

Salt and freshly ground black pepper

1 shallot, chopped

3 tablespoons very finely chopped fresh dill

6 teaspoons salmon roe

1 teaspoon crushed pink peppercorns

1 teaspoon ground dill seeds

1. Line six ¾-cup ramekins with plastic wrap.
2. Finely chop the tuna and the red snapper fillets.
3. Place the fish in a large bowl and toss with the vinegar and lime juice.
4. Season the mixture with salt and black pepper to taste, and add the shallot and fresh dill.
5. Divide the mixture equally among the prepared ramekins, pressing it down into the dishes.
6. Cover and refrigerate for 15 minutes.
7. Turn each ramekin out onto a dish.
8. Garnish each portion with a spoonful of salmon roe, and sprinkle with pink peppercorns and dill seeds.

Note: You will need six ¾-cup ramekins for this recipe. During the Cruise phase, you may serve this recipe with a slice of lime or on a bed of lettuce.

Note: Eating raw fish carries some risk of food-borne illness. Raw fish should not be consumed by the very young, the very old, pregnant women, or anyone with a compromised immune system.

Tuna Terrine

MAKES 2 SERVINGS
Preparation time: 15 minutes
Cooking time: 30 minutes

2 (5-ounce) cans of tuna packed in water, well drained
2 tablespoons fat-free plain Greek-style yogurt
2 eggs
Salt and freshly ground black pepper
1 teaspoon capers

1. Preheat oven to 350°F. Line a 9-inch loaf pan with nonstick foil or parchment paper.
2. In a medium bowl, combine one and a half cans of the tuna with the yogurt and eggs. Add salt and pepper to taste.
3. Stir until the mixture is smooth.
4. Add the remaining half can of tuna and the capers, and stir gently until combined.
5. Place the mixture in the prepared loaf pan and bake for 30 minutes.
6. Carefully invert the loaf pan onto a plate after baking and serve.

Note: You will need a 9-inch loaf pan for this recipe.

Spicy Tuna Salad

MAKES 3 SERVINGS
Preparation time: 10 minutes, plus 15 minutes for refrigeration
Cooking time: No cooking required

3 (5-ounce) cans of tuna packed in water
1 teaspoon chopped capers
1 tablespoon finely chopped onion
1 tablespoon finely chopped fresh parsley
¼ teaspoon curry powder
A few drops of Tabasco sauce

1. Drain the tuna, place in a medium bowl, and mix with the capers, onion, parsley, curry powder, and Tabasco.
2. Use a fork to break the tuna into slightly smaller pieces.
3. Cover and chill for at least 15 minutes before serving.

Tuna Carpaccio

MAKES 2 SERVINGS
Preparation time: 15 minutes
Cooking time: No cooking required

10 ounces Ahi tuna steaks
1 tablespoon low-sodium soy sauce
1 tablespoon fresh lemon juice
1 tablespoon tarragon vinegar
A few drops of Tabasco sauce
1 tablespoon chopped fresh herbs of your choice, such as
    parsley, sorrel, or chives
Salt

1. Freeze the tuna for 15 minutes, then cut into extremely thin strips, about ⅛ inch thick or thinner.
2. In a medium bowl, combine the soy sauce, lemon juice, tarragon vinegar, Tabasco, herbs, and salt to taste.
3. Brush the herb dressing on the fish and serve immediately.

Note: Eating raw fish carries some risk of food-borne illness. Raw fish should not be consumed by the very young, the very old, pregnant women, or anyone with a compromised immune system.
Note: During the Cruise phase, you may serve this recipe with lemon wedges.
Note: As a substitute for parsley, sorrel, or chives, you may use the same amount of spinach, with the addition of 1 teaspoon of lemon juice.

Grilled Tuna

MAKES 2 SERVINGS
Preparation time: 15 minutes
Cooking time: 10 minutes

2 tablespoons of very finely chopped fresh parsley
1 tablespoon of very finely chopped fresh oregano
1 tablespoon of very finely chopped fresh thyme
3 dried bay leaves, crushed
2 tablespoons fresh lemon juice
1 teaspoon mustard seeds
14 to 16 ounces tuna steaks, divided into two portions

1. Preheat oven to Broil for 5 minutes or heat a grill to high.
2. In a medium bowl, combine the parsley, oregano, thyme, bay leaves, lemon juice, and mustard seeds.
3. Brush the marinade all over each side of the steaks.
4. Broil or grill the fish until it is done to your liking, about 3 minutes on each side for medium-rare. While the steaks are cooking, brush them with some extra herb mixture.

Note: In the Cruise phase, you can serve this recipe with a warm tomato sauce.

Savory Tuna Bread

MAKES 2 SERVINGS
Preparation time: 10 minutes
Cooking time: 30 minutes

2 teaspoons active dry yeast
½ cup fat-free milk
2 (5-ounce) cans of tuna packed in water
1 tablespoon cornstarch (see Note)
3 eggs, beaten
Salt and freshly ground black pepper
⅛ teaspoon vegetable oil

1. Preheat oven to 400°F.
2. In a small bowl, combine the yeast and milk and stir until yeast is dissolved.
3. Chop up the tuna with a knife, place in a medium bowl, and combine with the cornstarch, eggs, and the milk mixture. Add salt and pepper to taste.
4. Add the oil to a 9-inch loaf pan, using a paper towel to coat it and to wipe out any excess.
5. Pour the mixture into the loaf pan and bake for 30 minutes.
6. Let cool, then turn the pan over to remove the bread before carefully slicing it to serve.

Note: You may eat this bread on pure protein days during the Cruise phase, not during the Attack phase. You may serve it with Dukan Mayonnaise (page 331) or a tomato sauce.

Seafood Loaf with Herbs

MAKES 2 SERVING
Preparation time: 10 minutes
Cooking time: 25 minutes

3 eggs, separated
6 tablespoons fat-free ricotta
1 tablespoon cornstarch
1 garlic clove, crushed
1 tablespoon finely chopped fresh herbs, such as parsley or chives
5 ounces fish fillets, such as cod or flounder, chopped
3 surimi (crab sticks), cut into thin slices, or 3 ounces crabmeat
Salt and freshly ground black pepper

1. Preheat oven to 350°F. Line a 9-inch loaf pan with foil or parchment paper.
2. In a mixing bowl, beat the egg whites until stiff.
3. Place the egg yolks in a large bowl and mix in the ricotta, cornstarch, garlic, and herbs.

4. Gently fold in the stiff egg whites.
5. Gently mix in the fish and the seafood sticks and season with salt and pepper to taste.
6. Place the mixture into the prepared loaf pan.
7. Bake for 25 minutes.
8. Let cool, then invert the loaf pan onto a plate and serve.

Note: You will need a 9-inch loaf pan for this recipe.
Note: You may eat this dish only on pure protein days during the Cruise phase, not during the Attack phase.

 Galettes ---

Dukan Oat Bran Galette

This light and easy pancake is a tasty way to eat your oat bran.

MAKES 1 GALETTE
Preparation time: 10 minutes
Cooking time: 10 minutes

2 tablespoons oat bran, such as Dukan Diet Organic Oat Bran
2 tablespoons fat-free plain Greek-style yogurt
1 teaspoon zero-calorie sweetener suited for cooking and
    baking, such as Splenda, for a sweet pancake
or
Freshly ground black pepper, fresh herbs, and/or chopped garlic
    for a savory pancake
1 egg white

1. In a medium bowl, combine the oat bran and yogurt with the sweetener for a sweet pancake, *or* with the pepper, herbs, and/or garlic for a savory pancake.
2. In a separate bowl, beat the egg white until foamy.
3. Fold the beaten egg white into the oat bran mixture until blended.
4. Heat a small nonstick pan over medium heat. Pour the

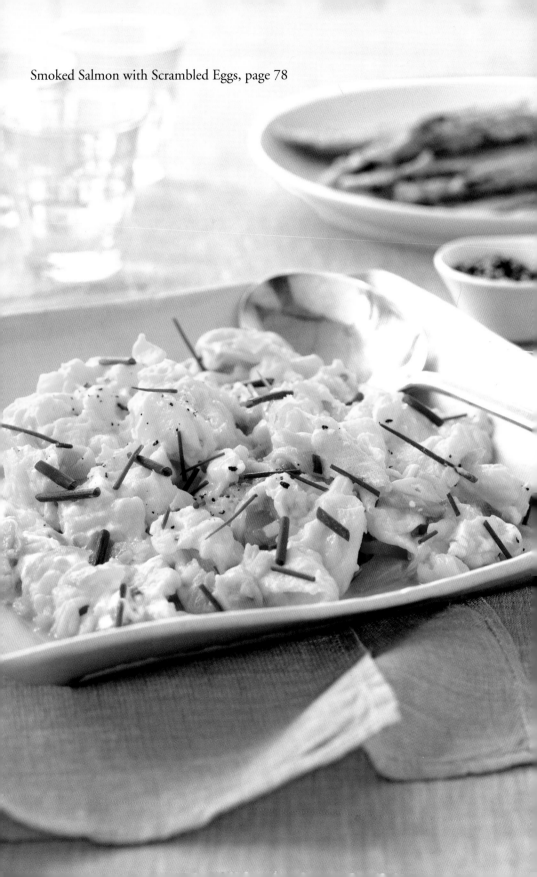

Smoked Salmon with Scrambled Eggs, page 78

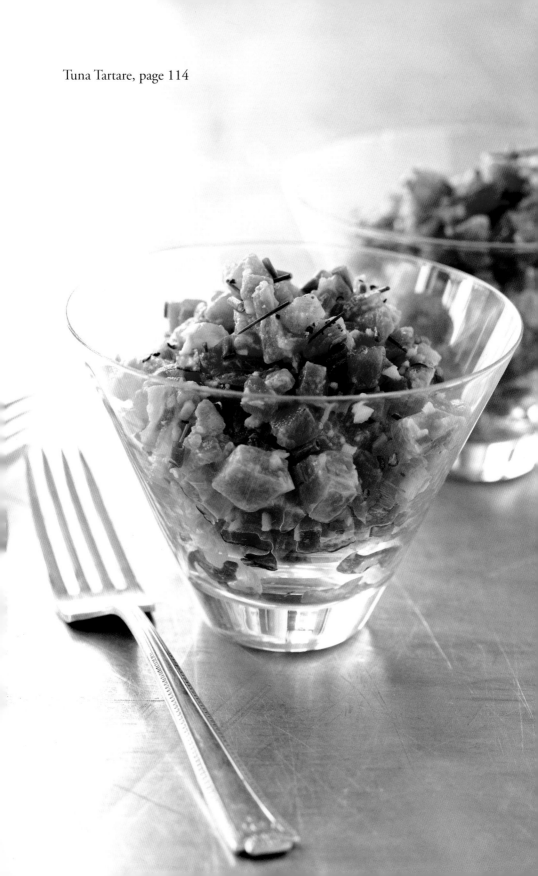

Tuna Tartare, page 114

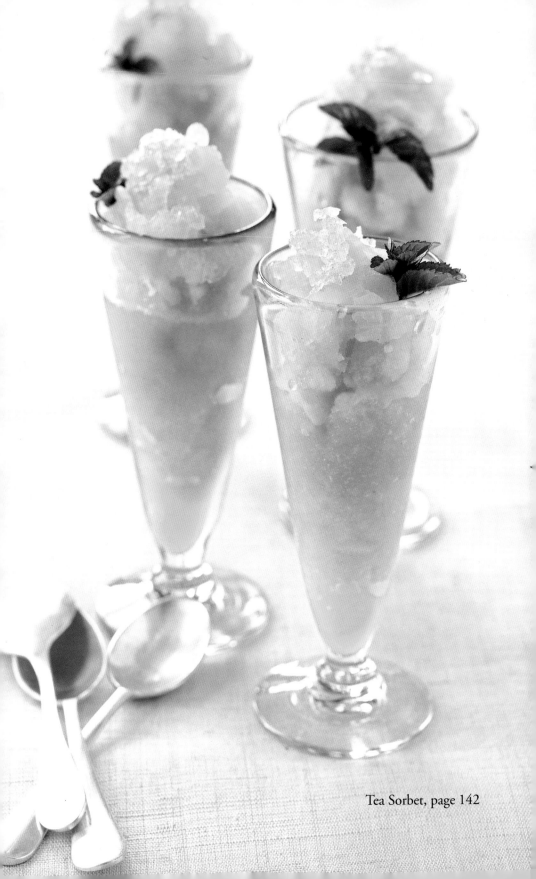

Tea Sorbet, page 142

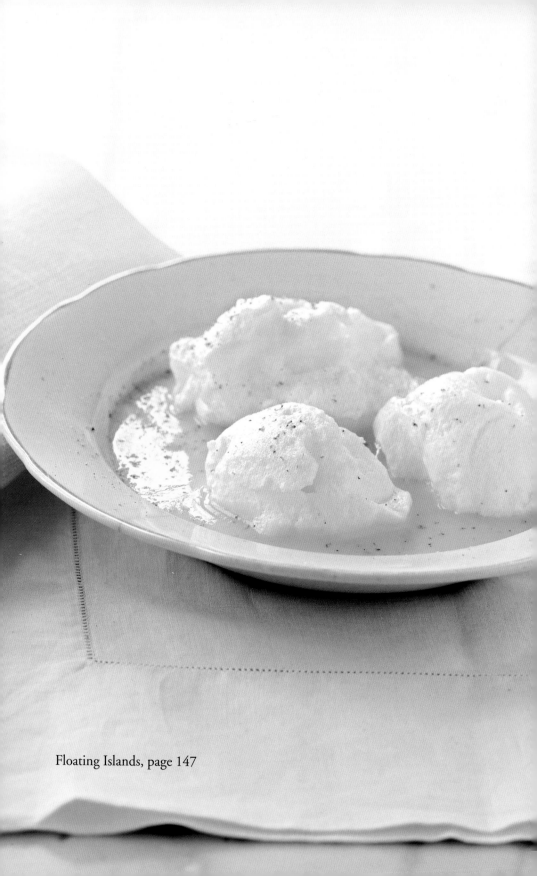

Floating Islands, page 147

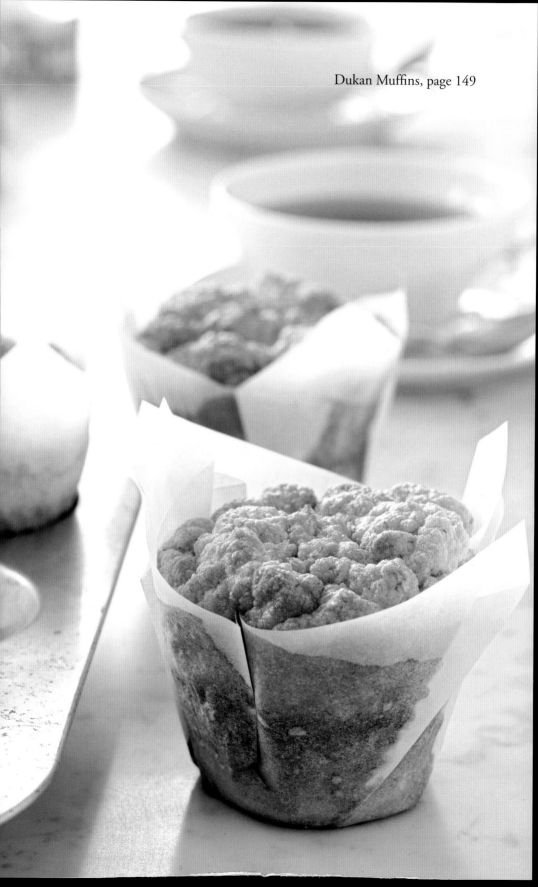
Dukan Muffins, page 149

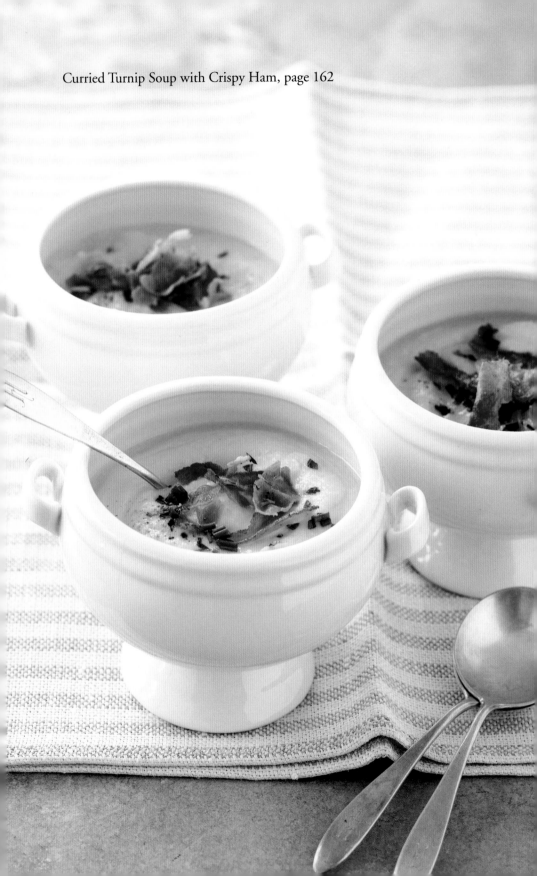

Curried Turnip Soup with Crispy Ham, page 162

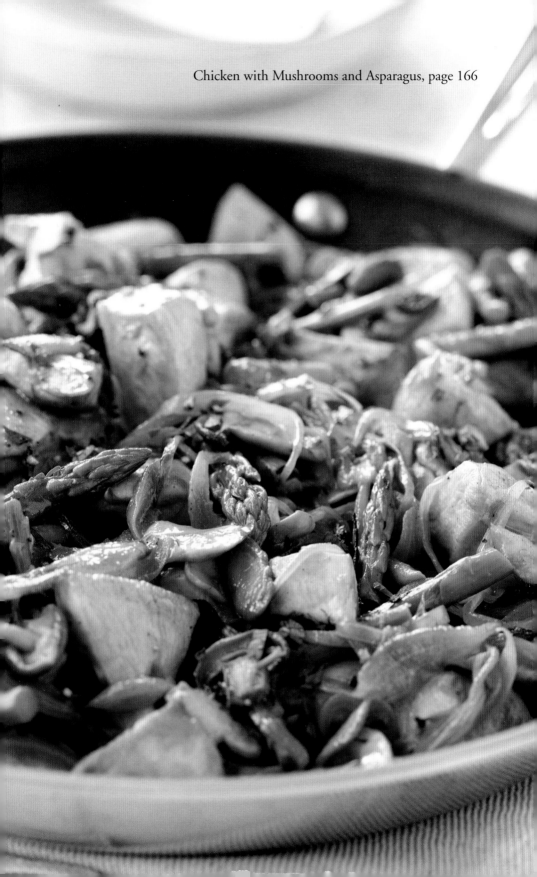

Chicken with Mushrooms and Asparagus, page 166

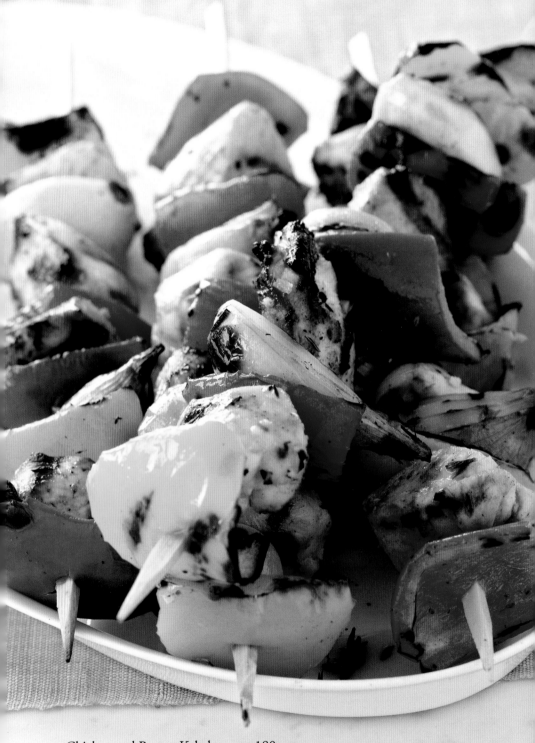

Chicken and Pepper Kebabs, page 180

mixture into the hot pan and cook until the underside is golden and the upper side starts to dry, about 3 minutes.

5. Using a spatula, flip the galette and continue cooking the other side until browned, about 2 more minutes.

6. Remove the galette to a plate and allow to cool briefly before serving.

Savory Galette

MAKES 2 SERVINGS

Preparation time: 20 minutes

Cooking time: 10 minutes

2 tablespoons oat bran, such as Dukan Diet Organic Oat Bran

1 tablespoon fat-free plain Greek-style yogurt

3 tablespoons fat-free ricotta

3 eggs, separated

1 tablespoon chopped fresh herbs, such as parsley, thyme, and sorrel

Salt and freshly ground black pepper

5 ounces tuna packed in water, drained, and flaked; *or* 7 ounces smoked salmon, chopped; *or* 5½ ounces extra-lean ham, chopped

1. In a large bowl, mix the oat bran, yogurt, ricotta, egg yolks, and herbs until smooth. Mix in salt and pepper to taste.

2. Add the protein of your choice and mix until combined.

3. In a medium bowl, beat the egg whites until stiff.

4. Fold the egg whites into the oat bran mixture.

5. Heat a medium nonstick frying pan over medium heat.

6. Pour the mixture into the hot pan and cook until browned on one side, about 3 minutes.

7. Using a spatula, flip the galette and continue cooking the other side until browned, about 2 more minutes.

Note: As a substitute for sorrel, you may use the same amount of spinach, with the addition of 1 teaspoon of lemon juice.

Sweet Galette

MAKES 1 SERVING

Preparation time: 20 minutes

Cooking time: 10 minutes

2 tablespoons oat bran, such as Dukan Diet Organic Oat Bran

1 tablespoon fat-free plain Greek-style yogurt

3 tablespoons fat-free ricotta

1 tablespoon zero-calorie sweetener suited for cooking and baking, such as Splenda

3 eggs, separated

1 teaspoon almond extract, *or* 1 teaspoon orange flower water, *or* 1 teaspoon unsweetened low-fat cocoa powder, such as Dukan Diet Organic Cocoa Powder

1. In a large bowl, mix together the oat bran, yogurt, ricotta, sweetener, egg yolks, and flavoring of your choice. (If flavoring with cocoa, do not add the cocoa now.)
2. In a mixing bowl, beat the egg whites until stiff.
3. Fold the egg whites into oat bran mixture.
4. Heat a medium nonstick frying pan over medium heat.
5. Pour the mixture into the hot pan and cook until browned on one side, about 3 minutes.
6. Using a spatula, flip the galette and continue cooking on the other side until browned, about 2 more minutes.
7. If making a chocolate galette, sift the cocoa powder on top of the galette before serving.

Bresaola Galette

MAKES 1 SERVING
Preparation time: 20 minutes
Cooking time: 10 minutes

2 tablespoons oat bran, such as Dukan Diet Organic Oat Bran

1 tablespoon fat-free plain Greek-style yogurt

3 tablespoons fat-free ricotta

3 eggs, separated

1 tablespoon chopped fresh herbs, such as parsley, oregano,
  and rosemary

Salt and freshly ground black pepper

2 ounces cooked bresaola sliced into thin strips (see Note)

1 tablespoon fat-free cottage cheese (optional)

1. In a large bowl, mix together the oat bran, yogurt, ricotta, egg yolks, and herbs. Add salt and pepper to taste.
2. In a mixing bowl, beat the egg whites until stiff.
3. Fold the egg whites into the oat bran mixture.
4. Heat a medium nonstick frying pan over medium heat.
5. Pour the mixture into the hot pan and cook until browned on one side, about 3 minutes.
6. Using a spatula, flip the galette and continue cooking on the other side until browned, about 2 more minutes.
7. To serve, top the galette with bresaola slices and fat-free cottage cheese (if desired).

Note: If bresaola is not available, you may substitute cooked turkey bacon.

Dukan Bread

MAKES 1 SERVING

Preparation time: 5 minutes

Cooking time: 10 minutes

1 tablespoon fat-free plain Greek-style yogurt

1 teaspoon active dry yeast

1 egg, beaten

1 tablespoon fat-free ricotta

1 tablespoon cornstarch (see Note)

1 teaspoon dried herbs and spices of your choice

1. Preheat oven to 400°F. You can also prepare this recipe in a microwave oven (see Note).
2. In a medium bowl, combine the yogurt and yeast. Stir until yeast is dissolved.
3. Add the egg, ricotta, cornstarch, and herbs, and mix until thoroughly combined.
4. Pour into a 6 × 8-inch nonstick baking pan that is at least ¼ inch deep.
5. Bake in the oven until set, about 10 minutes.
6. Once the bread is cooked, immediately turn it out of the pan and place it on a cooling rack. Slice the bread and use it to make roast turkey or smoked salmon sandwiches.

Note: If using a microwave, place the bread in a microwave-safe pan, and cook on the highest setting for 5 minutes. As soon as the bread is ready, turn the loaf out from the pan, and place it on a cooling rack.
Note: You may eat this bread only on pure protein days during the Cruise phase, not during the Attack phase.

Cinnamon Tart

MAKES 4 SERVINGS
Preparation time: 25 minutes
Cooking time: 40 minutes

2 tablespoons oat bran, such as Dukan Diet Organic Oat Bran
1 tablespoon fat-free plain Greek-style yogurt
3 tablespoons fat-free ricotta
1 teaspoon zero-calorie sweetener suited for cooking and
    baking, such as Splenda
3 eggs, separated

FOR THE TOPPING
3 eggs
1 tablespoon zero-calorie sweetener suited for cooking and
    baking, such as Splenda
½ cup fat-free plain Greek-style yogurt
½ cup fat-free ricotta
1 teaspoon cinnamon
Seeds from 1 vanilla bean, or ¼ teaspoon vanilla extract

1. Preheat oven to 325°F.
2. In a large bowl, mix together the oat bran, yogurt, ricotta, sweetener, and egg yolks.
3. In a mixing bowl, beat the egg whites until stiff.
4. Fold the egg whites into the oat bran mixture.
5. Line a 9-inch cake pan with wax paper or parchment paper.
6. Pour the mixture into the prepared pan and bake for 10 minutes.
7. While the crust is baking, make the topping.
8. In a medium bowl, beat the 3 whole eggs, add the sweetener, and continue beating until the mixture is thick.
9. Mix in the yogurt, ricotta, cinnamon, and vanilla until smooth.
10. Once the crust is baked, pour the topping on top and bake for an additional 30 minutes.

Breakfast Oat Bran Muesli

MAKES 4 SERVINGS

Preparation time: 5 minutes

Cooking time: 30 minutes

6 tablespoons oat bran, such as Dukan Diet Organic Oat Bran

1 egg white

¼ teaspoon stevia, such as Dukan Diet Organic Stevia

½ teaspoon almond extract

1 tablespoon flax seed or chia seed (optional)

1. Preheat oven to 325°F.
2. Combine all ingredients in a medium bowl.
3. Place a piece of parchment on a baking sheet, and spread out oat bran mix.
4. Bake for 30 minutes, or until golden brown.
5. Allow to cool, then crumble and store in an airtight container. Add to yogurt or enjoy a portion of the muesli with some Goji berries for a healthy snack.

Discover Dukan Diet Organic Cocoa Powder

Discover Dukan Diet Organic Oat Bran

Discover Dukan Diet Organic Stevia

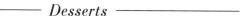

Desserts

Some of these recipes contain raw or undercooked eggs. Raw or under-cooked eggs should not be consumed by the very young, the very old, pregnant women, or anyone with a compromised immune system.

Vanilla Bavarian Cream

MAKES 2 SERVINGS

Preparation time: 15 minutes, plus overnight refrigeration

Cooking time: No cooking required

1½ (7-gram) envelopes (10½ grams total) of unflavored gelatin
2 cups cold fat-free vanilla-flavored Greek-style yogurt
2 egg whites
1 tablespoon zero-calorie sweetener suited for cooking and
    baking, such as Splenda

1. In a medium bowl, combine the gelatin and 3 tablespoons of the yogurt, and let sit for 5 minutes.
2. Meanwhile, in a medium mixing bowl, beat the egg whites until stiff.
3. Add 3 tablespoons of hot water to the gelatin and yogurt mixture and stir until smooth.
4. In a mixing bowl, whip the remaining yogurt until light and smooth, about 2 minutes, then add the stiff egg whites and the gelatin and yogurt mixture.
5. Continue beating the mixture for 2 to 3 minutes.
6. Add the sweetener, place in a nonreactive bowl, cover, and refrigerate overnight. Serve cold.

Almond Milk Jellies

MAKES 2 SERVINGS

Preparation time: 15 minutes, plus 1 hour for refrigeration

Cooking time: 5 minutes

1½ (7-gram) envelopes (10½ grams total) of unflavored gelatin

1¾ cups cold fat-free milk

½ teaspoon almond extract

2 teaspoons zero-calorie sweetener suited for cooking and
baking, such as Splenda

1. In a medium bowl, combine the gelatin and ¼ cup of the cold milk.
2. In a saucepan, heat the remaining milk, add the almond extract, the sweetener, and bring to a boil.
3. Add the gelatin mixture to the hot milk mixture and stir until the gelatin has completely dissolved.
4. Pour the mixture into a 9-inch-square nonstick pan, cover, and refrigerate until set, about 1 hour. To serve, cut into bite-sized squares.

Blancmange

MAKES 2 SERVINGS

Preparation time: 25 minutes, plus 2 hours for refrigeration

Cooking time: 5 minutes

1 (7-gram) envelope of unflavored gelatin

1¾ cups fat-free plain Greek-style yogurt

2 teaspoons zero-calorie sweetener suited for cooking and
baking, such as Splenda

¼ teaspoon almond extract

1 egg white

1. In a medium bowl, combine the gelatin and ½ cup of the yogurt. Let sit for 5 minutes.

2. In a small saucepan, warm another ¼ cup of the yogurt over low heat.

3. Combine the gelatin mixture with the warm yogurt and stir until the gelatin is completely dissolved.

4. In a large bowl, combine the remaining 1 cup of yogurt, the gelatin mixture, 1 teaspoon of the sweetener, and the almond extract.

5. In a medium bowl beat the egg white until soft peaks form. Add the remaining sweetener and continue beating until stiff.

6. Gently fold the egg white into the yogurt mixture.

7. Divide the mixture equally among two 1-cup ramekins, cover, and refrigerate for at least 2 hours before serving.

Note: You will need two 1-cup ramekins for this recipe.

Note: Raw or undercooked eggs should not be consumed by the very young, the very old, pregnant women, or anyone with a compromised immune system.

Cheesecake

MAKES 2 SERVINGS

Preparation time: 10 minutes, plus 2 hours for refrigeration
Cooking time: 12 minutes

⅛ teaspoon vegetable oil

5 tablespoons fat-free plain Greek-style yogurt

2 tablespoons cornstarch (see Note)

2 egg yolks

2 tablespoons fresh lemon juice

2 teaspoons zero-calorie sweetener suited for cooking and baking, such as Splenda

5 egg whites

1. Add the oil to a 2-cup soufflé dish and use a paper towel to wipe out any excess.

2. In a medium bowl, beat together the yogurt, cornstarch, egg yolks, lemon juice, and sweetener until the mixture is frothy.

3. In a medium bowl, beat the egg whites until stiff, then carefully fold them into the yogurt mixture.
4. Pour the mixture into the prepared soufflé dish.
5. Microwave for 12 minutes on medium power. Cover and refrigerate for at least 2 hours. Serve cold.

Note: You may eat this cheesecake only on pure protein days during the Cruise phase, not during the Attack phase.

Vanilla Cookie

MAKES 1 SERVING
Preparation time: 10 minutes
Cooking time: 20 minutes

⅛ teaspoon vegetable oil
2 eggs, separated
½ teaspoon zero-calorie sweetener suited for cooking and baking, such as Splenda
½ teaspoon vanilla extract
2 tablespoons oat bran, such as Dukan Diet Organic Oat Bran (see Note)

1. Preheat oven to 350°F.
2. Line a baking sheet with parchment paper and coat the paper with the oil.
3. In a medium bowl, mix the egg yolks, sweetener, vanilla, and oat bran until thoroughly combined.
4. In a medium mixing bowl, beat the egg whites until very stiff. Carefully fold them into the bran mixture.
5. Pour the mixture onto the prepared baking sheet and bake until golden brown, about 15 to 20 minutes.

Note: You may eat this cookie only on pure protein days during the Cruise phase. You can reduce the oat bran amount to 1½ tablespoons during the Attack phase.

Coffee Custard

MAKES 4 SERVINGS

Preparation time: 5 minutes

Cooking time: 45 minutes plus at least 3 hours for refrigeration

⅛ teaspoon vegetable oil

2 cups fat-free milk

1 teaspoon instant coffee

3 eggs

2 egg yolks

1 tablespoon zero-calorie sweetener suited for cooking and
baking, such as Splenda

1. Preheat oven to 325°F.
2. Distribute the oil among four ¾-cup ramekins, using a paper towel to coat them and to wipe out any excess.
3. In a saucepan, combine the milk and instant coffee, bring to a boil, and stir until the coffee is completely dissolved.
4. In a mixing bowl, beat the whole eggs, yolks, and sweetener.
5. Gradually add the milk and coffee mixture to the eggs, stirring continuously.
6. Pour the mixture into the prepared ramekins, place the ramekins into a large baking dish, and fill the dish halfway with cold water.
7. Place the baking dish in the oven, and bake the custard for 40 minutes or until set. Cool, cover, and refrigerate for at least 3 hours. Serve cold.

Note: You will need four ¾-cup ramekins for this recipe.

Spiced Custard

MAKES 2 SERVINGS

Preparation time: 20 minutes, plus 1 hour for refrigeration

Cooking time: 20 minutes

1 cup fat-free milk

1 vanilla bean, split in half lengthways, or ¼ teaspoon vanilla
extract

½ teaspoon ground cinnamon

1 clove

1 star anise

2 egg yolks

2 teaspoons zero-calorie sweetener suited for cooking and
baking, such as Splenda

1 cup fat-free plain Greek-style yogurt

1. In a medium saucepan, combine the milk, vanilla, cinnamon, clove, and star anise and bring to a boil.
2. In a medium bowl, beat the egg yolks and the sweetener until the mixture turns pale.
3. Gradually pour the hot milk over the egg mixture, stirring continuously.
4. Pour the mixture back into the saucepan and cook for 12 minutes over gentle heat, stirring frequently until the cream coats a spoon.
5. Strain the custard and allow it to cool.
6. Once the custard is cool, mix in the yogurt until thoroughly combined.
7. Cover and refrigerate for at least 1 hour. Serve cold.

Vanilla Custard

MAKES 2 SERVINGS

Preparation time: 15 minutes

Cooking time: 30 minutes

⅛ teaspoon vegetable oil

2¼ cups fat-free milk

3 eggs

2 egg yolks

2 teaspoons zero-calorie sweetener suited for cooking and
baking, such as Splenda

⅛ teaspoon vanilla extract

A pinch of grated nutmeg

1. Preheat oven to 350°F.
2. Add the oil to a 4-cup baking dish, using a paper towel to coat it and to wipe out any excess.
3. Whisk together the milk, whole eggs, egg yolks, sweetener, and vanilla.
4. Pour this mixture into the prepared baking dish and sprinkle with nutmeg.
5. Place the baking dish into a bigger dish and fill the larger dish halfway with cold water.
6. Place in the oven and bake for 30 minutes, until the custard is firm to the touch.
7. Serve warm or cold.

Dukan Whipped Crème

MAKES 1 SERVING

Preparation time: 5 minutes, plus 3 hours for refrigeration
Cooking time: No cooking required

¼ cup fat-free plain Greek-style yogurt
5 tablespoons fat-free ricotta
1½ teaspoons zero-calorie sweetener suited for cooking and
    baking, such as Splenda
2 egg whites or 2 pasteurized egg whites

1. In a small bowl, beat the yogurt, ricotta, and sweetener.
2. In a medium mixing bowl, beat the egg whites until stiff.
3. Gently fold the egg whites into the yogurt mixture.
4. Cover and refrigerate for at least 3 hours. Serve cold.

Note: Raw or undercooked eggs should not be consumed by the very young, the very old, pregnant women, or anyone with a compromised immune system.

Coffee Pudding

MAKES 1 SERVING

Preparation time: 5 minutes, plus 1 hour for refrigeration
Cooking time: 5 minutes

½ cup fat-free milk
A pinch of instant coffee
1 teaspoon zero-calorie sweetener suited for cooking and
    baking, such as Splenda
½ (7-gram) envelope (3½ grams or 1 teaspoon total) of
    unflavored powdered gelatin

1. Place the milk, coffee, and sweetener in a saucepan and heat until hot. Do not boil.
2. In a small bowl, combine the gelatin and 3 tablespoons of cold water. Let sit for 5 minutes.

3. Add the gelatin to the milk mixture and mix until thoroughly combined.

4. Pour the mixture into a 1-cup dish or ramekin, cover, and refrigerate until set, about 1 hour.

Dukan Crème Brûlée

MAKES 2 SERVINGS

Preparation time: 15 minutes

Cooking time: 25 minutes

⅛ teaspoon vegetable oil

2 eggs, separated

6 tablespoons fat-free plain Greek-style yogurt

1 tablespoon zero-calorie sweetener suited for cooking and baking, such as Splenda

1 teaspoon lemon juice or orange flower water

1. Preheat oven to 350°F.

2. Distribute the oil between two 1-cup ramekins, using a paper towel to coat them and to wipe out any excess.

3. In a medium bowl whisk the egg yolks, yogurt, sweetener, and lemon juice until smooth.

4. In a medium bowl, beat the egg whites until stiff.

5. Gently fold the egg whites into the egg yolk mixture.

6. Pour the egg mixture into the prepared ramekin dishes and bake for 20 minutes. Turn the oven to Broil and cook until the tops are browned, about 5 minutes.

Note: You will need two 1-cup ramekins for this recipe.

Lemon Mousse

MAKES 4 SERVINGS

Preparation time: 15 minutes, plus 1 hour for refrigeration

Cooking time: No cooking required

1¼ cups fat-free plain Greek-style yogurt

1½ (7-gram) envelopes (10½ grams or 1 tablespoon total) of unflavored gelatin

2 tablespoons fresh lemon juice

2 eggs, separated

2 teaspoons zero-calorie sweetener suited for cooking and baking, such as Splenda, to taste

1. In a medium bowl, combine 2 tablespoons of the yogurt with the gelatin. Let sit for 5 minutes.
2. In a saucepan, warm the lemon juice over low heat.
3. Add the lemon juice to the gelatin mixture and stir until the gelatin is completely dissolved.
4. In a medium bowl, combine the remaining yogurt, egg yolks, and sweetener. Add the gelatin mixture.
5. In a medium bowl, beat the egg whites until stiff.
6. Gently fold the egg whites into the lemon mixture, place in a 2-cup bowl, cover, and refrigerate until set, about 1 hour.

Note: Raw or undercooked eggs should not be consumed by the very young, the very old, pregnant women, or anyone with a compromised immune system.

Flan

MAKES 4 SERVINGS
Preparation time: 15 minutes
Cooking time: 35 minutes

⅛ teaspoon vegetable oil

5 eggs

1½ cups fat-free milk

1 vanilla bean, split in half lengthways or 1 teaspoon vanilla
   extract

2 teaspoons zero-calorie sweetener suited for cooking and
   baking, such as Splenda

A pinch of ground nutmeg

1. Preheat oven to 375°F.
2. Distribute the oil among four ¾-cup ramekins, using a paper towel to coat them and to wipe out any excess.
3. In a large bowl, beat the eggs.
4. In a small saucepan, combine the milk and the vanilla and heat until hot. Do not boil.
5. Gradually pour the hot milk over the eggs, whisking constantly. Add the sweetener and nutmeg.
6. Pour the mixture into the prepared ramekin dishes and bake until set, about 30 minutes.
7. To serve, let cool, and turn out of the ramekins.

Note: You will need four ¾-cup ramekins for this recipe.

Lemon Cheesecake

MAKES 4 SERVINGS

Preparation time: 10 minutes

Cooking time: 20 minutes

⅛ teaspoon vegetable oil

½ cup fat-free plain Greek-style yogurt

1 teaspoon active dry yeast

2 tablespoons cornstarch (see Note)

Grated zest of 1 lemon

2 teaspoons zero-calorie sweetener suited for cooking and
   baking, such as Splenda

2 egg yolks

4 egg whites

1. Preheat oven to 400°F.
2. Add the oil to an 8-inch round cake pan, using a paper towel to coat it and to wipe out any excess.
3. In a large bowl, mix together the yogurt and yeast. Let sit for 5 minutes, then stir until yeast is dissolved.
4. Add the cornstarch, lemon zest, sweetener, and egg yolks to the yogurt mixture and mix until combined.
5. In a medium mixing bowl, beat the egg whites until stiff.
6. Fold the egg whites into the yogurt mixture.
7. Pour the batter into the prepared pan and bake for 20 minutes. Serve at room temperature.

Note: You may eat this cheesecake only on pure protein days during the Cruise phase, not during the Attack phase.

Yogurt Pudding

MAKES 4 SERVINGS

Preparation time: 15 minutes

Cooking time: 20 minutes

⅛ teaspoon vegetable oil

2 eggs, separated

1 tablespoon zero-calorie sweetener suited for cooking and
baking, such as Splenda

¾ cup fat-free plain Greek-style yogurt

3 tablespoons cornstarch (see Note)

1 teaspoon grated lemon zest, *or* ½ teaspoon ground cinnamon,
or ¼ teaspoon coffee extract

A pinch of salt

1. Preheat oven to 425°F.
2. Add the oil to an 8-inch round cake pan, using a paper towel to coat it and to wipe out any excess.
3. In a medium bowl, mix the egg yolks and sweetener until thoroughly combined.
4. Mix in the yogurt, cornstarch, and flavoring of your choice.
5. In a medium bowl, beat the egg whites with a pinch of salt until very stiff.
6. Gently fold the egg whites into the yogurt mixture.
7. Pour the batter into the prepared cake pan and bake for 20 minutes.

Note: You may eat this pudding only on pure protein days during the Cruise phase, not during the Attack phase.

Nana's Cake

MAKES 2 SERVINGS
Preparation time: 15 minutes
Cooking time: 25 minutes

⅛ teaspoon vegetable oil

2 heaping tablespoons cornstarch (see Note)

1½ teaspoons zero-calorie sweetener suited for cooking and
    baking, such as Splenda

Grated zest of 1 lemon

3 eggs, separated

3 heaping tablespoons fat-free plain Greek-style yogurt

1. Preheat oven to 350°F.
2. Add the oil to an 8-inch round cake pan, using a paper towel
   to coat it and to wipe out any excess.
3. In a medium bowl, mix the cornstarch, sweetener, lemon
   zest, egg yolks, and yogurt until thoroughly combined.
4. In a medium bowl, beat the egg whites until stiff.
5. Fold the egg whites into the yogurt mixture.
6. Pour the batter into the prepared pan and bake for 25 minutes.

Note: You may eat this cake only on pure protein days during the
Cruise phase, not during the Attack phase.

Sponge Cake

MAKES 2 SERVINGS
Preparation time: 10 minutes
Cooking time: 20 minutes

⅛ teaspoon vegetable oil

4 eggs, separated

2 teaspoons zero-calorie sweetener suited for cooking and
    baking, such as Splenda

Grated zest of 1 lemon

3 tablespoons cornstarch (see Note)

1. Preheat oven to 350°F.
2. Line a 9-inch round cake pan with parchment paper and coat the paper with the vegetable oil.
3. In a medium bowl, mix together the egg yolks and sweetener, then add the lemon zest and cornstarch.
4. In a medium mixing bowl, beat the egg whites until stiff.
5. Carefully fold the egg whites into the egg yolk mixture.
6. Place the batter into the prepared pan and bake until the cake is golden brown, about 20 minutes.

Note: You may eat this cake only on pure protein days during the Cruise phase, not during the Attack phase.

Coffee and Cinnamon Granita

MAKES 2 SERVINGS

Preparation time: 30 minutes, plus 1 hour freezing time

Cooking time: No cooking required

2¼ cups hot black coffee
2 teaspoons zero-calorie sweetener suited for cooking and baking, such as Splenda
1 teaspoon ground cinnamon
3 cardamom seeds

1. In a medium bowl, mix the hot coffee, sweetener, and spices.
2. Pour the mixture into a 9 × 13-inch metal pan and freeze uncovered for about 20 minutes.
3. Drag a fork through the top layer of ice crystals until the crystals flake. Return the pan to the freezer. Repeat every 20 to 30 minutes until the entire mixture is flaky.
4. Divide the granita between two dishes and serve.

Tea Sorbet

MAKES 2 SERVINGS

Preparation time: 20 minutes, plus 1 hour freezing time

Cooking time: No cooking required

3 tablespoons loose black tea

2 tablespoons fresh lemon juice

1½ teaspoons zero-calorie sweetener suited for cooking and
baking, such as Splenda

4 fresh mint leaves

1. In a medium bowl, combine 1¼ cups boiling water with the tea, cover, and leave to infuse for 3 minutes. Strain out the tea leaves.
2. Measure 4 tablespoons of the infused tea and pour it into a flat, freezer-proof dish.
3. Cover and freeze, stirring occasionally with a fork, until ice crystals start to form.
4. Add lemon juice and sweetener to the remaining tea infusion.
5. Pour the tea and lemon mixture into an ice cream machine and churn until frozen, about 15 minutes.
6. When ready to serve, fill glasses with the sorbet and top with the iced tea crystals (from step 3).
7. Garnish with the mint leaves.

Note: You will need an ice cream machine for this recipe.

Lime Sorbet

MAKES 2 TO 3 SERVINGS

Preparation time: 15 minutes, plus freezing time

Cooking time: No cooking required

Grated zest of 1 lime

¼ cup fresh lime juice

2¼ cups fat-free plain Greek-style yogurt

2 teaspoons zero-calorie sweetener suited for cooking and
    baking, such as Splenda

1. In a blender, combine the lime zest, lime juice, yogurt, and sweetener. Process until thoroughly combined, about 30 seconds.
2. Place the mixture in a bowl, cover, and refrigerate until cold.
3. Churn in an ice cream machine until frozen, about 15 minutes.

Note: You will need an ice cream machine for this recipe

Tart Frozen Yogurt

MAKES 2 TO 3 SERVINGS

Preparation time: 1 hour

Cooking time: No cooking required

1¼ cups plus 2 tablespoons fat-free plain Greek-style yogurt

Grated zest and juice of 2 lemons

1. In a blender, combine the yogurt, lemon zest, and lemon juice. Process until thoroughly combined, about 30 seconds.
2. Place the mixture in a bowl, cover, and refrigerate until cold.
3. Churn in an ice cream machine until frozen, about 15 minutes.

Note: You will need an ice cream machine for this recipe.

Salted Lassi

MAKES 4 SERVINGS

Preparation time: 5 minutes, plus 1 hour for refrigeration

Cooking time: No cooking required

2 cups fat-free plain Greek-style yogurt

2¼ cups fat-free milk

A pinch of salt

¼ teaspoon crushed green cardamom

⅛ teaspoon rose water

1. In a large bowl, combine the yogurt, milk, salt, cardamom, and rose water. Whisk until thoroughly combined.
2. Cover, refrigerate for 1 hour, and serve cold in glasses.

Coffee Mousse

MAKES 4 SERVINGS

Preparation time: 10 minutes, plus 3 hours for refrigeration

Cooking time: No cooking required

⅓ cup fat-free plain Greek-style yogurt

½ cup fat-free ricotta

2 tablespoons zero-calorie sweetener suited for cooking and baking, such as Splenda

1 tablespoon coffee extract

4 egg whites

1. In a large bowl, whisk the yogurt and ricotta until light and fluffy, then add the sweetener and coffee extract and mix until thoroughly combined.
2. In a medium mixing bowl, beat the egg whites until stiff, then carefully fold them into the yogurt mixture.
3. Spoon the mixture into four ½-cup ramekins, cover, and refrigerate for 3 hours before serving.

Note: You will need four ½-cup ramekins for this recipe.

Note: Raw or undercooked eggs should not be consumed by the very young, the very old, pregnant women, or anyone with a compromised immune system.

Lemon Mousse

MAKES 2 SERVINGS

Preparation time: 20 minutes, plus 2 hours for refrigeration

Cooking time: 2 minutes

1 cup fat-free plain Greek-style yogurt

1 (7-gram) envelope of unflavored powdered gelatin

2 teaspoons zero-calorie sweetener suited for cooking and baking, such as Splenda

Grated zest of ½ lemon

1 egg, separated

1. In a small bowl, combine 2 tablespoons of the yogurt with the gelatin. Let sit for 5 minutes.
2. In a medium bowl, combine the sweetener, lemon zest, ¼ cup of the yogurt, and the egg yolk.
3. Whisk together until the mixture is smooth and light yellow in color.
4. Pour the mixture into a small saucepan and warm over low heat for 2 minutes.
5. Mix in the gelatin mixture until the gelatin is completely dissolved.
6. Whisk in the remaining yogurt (½ cup plus 2 tablespoons).
7. In a mixing bowl, beat the egg white until stiff.
8. Gently fold the beaten egg white into the lemon cream.
9. Cover and refrigerate for 2 hours, or until set.

Note: Raw or undercooked eggs should not be consumed by the very young, the very old, pregnant women, or anyone with a compromised immune system.

Cinnamon Mousse

MAKES 4 SERVINGS

Preparation time: 15 minutes, plus 2 hours for refrigeration

Cooking time: No cooking required

2½ cups fat-free plain Greek-style yogurt

4 eggs, separated

1 teaspoon ground cinnamon

1 tablepoon zero-calorie sweetener suited for cooking and
baking, such as Splenda

1. In a medium bowl, beat together the egg yolks and the yogurt, then add the cinnamon and sweetener.
2. In a medium mixing bowl, beat the egg whites until stiff.
3. Gently fold the stiffly beaten egg whites into the yogurt mixture.
4. Cover and refrigerate for 2 hours, or until set.

Note: Raw or undercooked eggs should not be consumed by the very young, the very old, pregnant women, or anyone with a compromised immune system.

Iced Lemon Mousse

MAKES 2 TO 3 SERVINGS

Preparation time: 10 minutes, plus 2 hours for freezing

Cooking time: No cooking required

2¼ cups fat-free plain Greek-style yogurt

2 teaspoons zero-calorie sweetener suited for cooking and
baking, such as Splenda

Grated zest of 1 lemon

¾ cup fresh lemon juice

4 egg whites

1. In a medium bowl, whisk the yogurt, then add the lemon zest and lemon juice.

2. In a mixing bowl, beat the egg whites until stiff.
3. Carefully fold the egg whites into the yogurt mixture.
4. Place the mousse in a freezer-proof dish, cover, and freeze for 2 hours or until firm.

Note: Raw or undercooked eggs should not be consumed by the very young, the very old, pregnant women, or anyone with a compromised immune system.

Floating Islands

MAKES 2 SERVINGS

Preparation time: 20 minutes, plus 3 hours for refrigeration
Cooking time: 15 minutes

1 cup fat-free milk
2 eggs, separated
1 tablespoon zero-calorie sweetener suited for cooking and
    baking, such as Splenda

1. Cover a large plate with cheesecloth.
2. To make the custard, pour the milk into a saucepan and bring to a boil.
3. In a medium bowl, beat the egg yolks and mix in the sweetener.
4. Gradually mix in the boiling milk, stirring continuously.
5. Pour the mixture back into the saucepan and warm over low heat, stirring constantly with a wooden spoon and making sure that none of the mixture sticks to the bottom of the pan. Do not let the mixture boil.
6. As soon as the custard starts to thicken, remove the saucepan from the heat and pour it into a bowl.
7. To make the meringues, fill a large saucepan with water and bring to a boil.
8. In a medium bowl, beat the egg whites until stiff.
9. Using a tablespoon, drop dollops of egg white into the boiling water.

10. As soon as the egg whites start to swell up, remove them with a slotted spoon, place them on cheesecloth, and leave them to drain.

11. Once the custard has completely cooled to room temperature, arrange the meringues on top.

12. Cover and refrigerate for 3 hours. Serve chilled.

Note: You will need cheesecloth for this recipe.

Egg Custard

MAKES 2 SERVINGS

Preparation time: 10 minutes

Cooking time: 50 minutes

⅛ teaspoon vegetable oil

1 vanilla bean, split in half lengthwise

1¼ cups fat-free milk

2 tablespoons zero-calorie sweetener suited for cooking and baking, such as Splenda

4 eggs

1. Preheat oven to 425°F.

2. Add the oil to a 4-cup baking dish, using a paper towel to coat it and to wipe out any excess.

3. In a medium saucepan, add the vanilla bean, milk, and sweetener and bring to a boil. Once the milk boils, remove the vanilla bean and discard it.

4. In a medium bowl, whisk the eggs, and gradually pour the hot milk over the beaten eggs, stirring constantly.

5. Pour the mixture into the prepared baking dish.

6. Place the dish inside a larger dish and fill this larger dish halfway with cold water.

7. Bake for 40 minutes. Cool, cover, and refrigerate until ready to serve.

Dukan Muffins

MAKES 4 SERVINGS

Preparation time: 10 minutes

Cooking time: 25 minutes

4 eggs, separated

½ cup oat bran, such as Dukan Diet Organic Oat Bran

¼ cup fat-free plain Greek-style yogurt

½ teaspoon zero-calorie sweetener suited for cooking and
baking, such as Splenda

2 teaspoons grated lemon zest *or* ½ teaspoon ground cinnamon
or ¼ teaspoon coffee extract

1. Preheat oven to 350°F.
2. In a medium bowl, mix the egg yolks, oat bran, yogurt, sweetener, and flavoring of your choice until thoroughly combined.
3. In a medium mixing bowl, beat the egg whites until stiff.
4. Gently fold the egg whites into the oat bran mixture.
5. Spoon the batter into a nonstick or silicon muffin tin and bake until cooked through, about 25 minutes.

Note: If your muffin tin holds more than 4 muffins, fill the empty spaces with water to prevent the tins from burning.

Lemon "Tart"

MAKES 3 SERVINGS
Preparation time: 15 minutes
Cooking time: 30 minutes

⅛ teaspoon vegetable oil

3 eggs, separated

1 tablespoon zero-calorie sweetener suited for cooking and
baking, such as Splenda, divided

Grated zest and juice of 1 lemon

A pinch of salt

1. Preheat oven to 350°F.
2. Add the oil to a nonstick 9-inch baking dish, using a paper towel to coat it and to wipe out any excess.
3. In a medium heatproof bowl, beat the egg yolks with a pinch of sweetener. Add 2 tablespoons of water and the lemon zest and juice.
4. Fill a medium saucepan halfway with water and bring it to a simmer.
5. Place the bowl containing the egg yolk mixture over the pot. The bottom of the bowl must not touch the water.
6. Cook over low heat, stirring the egg mixture constantly with a spatula, until the mixture thickens.
7. Remove the bowl from the heat and set it aside.
8. In a medium mixing bowl, beat the egg whites until stiff. Mix in the salt and the remaining sweetener.
9. Carefully fold the egg whites into the hot egg mixture.
10. Pour the mixture into the prepared baking dish.
11. Bake until golden brown on top, about 20 minutes.

Discover Dukan Diet Organic Oat Bran

Recipes with Proteins and Vegetables

Soups

Chilled Cucumber and Shrimp Soup

MAKES 4 SERVINGS

Preparation time: 30 minutes, plus 1 hour for chilling

Cooking time: No cooking required

2 small cucumbers, peeled and with seeds removed

1 onion, quartered

1 garlic clove

6 tablespoons fresh lemon juice

2 tablespoons anisette (aniseed-flavored liqueur) (optional)

Salt and freshly ground black pepper

4 sprigs of fresh cilantro, very finely chopped

8 large shrimp, cooked and shelled, with tails removed

A few drops of Tabasco sauce

¼ red bell pepper, with seeds removed and very thinly sliced

½ red onion, very thinly sliced

1. In a blender, process the cucumbers, onion, garlic, 3 tablespoons of the lemon juice, and the anisette (if using), along with salt and pepper to taste.

2. Add 2 cups of spring water and half the cilantro. Blend until smooth, about 30 seconds.

3. Pour the soup into a medium container, cover, and place in the refrigerator for one hour.

4. Half an hour before you are ready to serve the soup, split the shrimp lengthwise and spread them out on a plate.

5. Dress the shrimp with the remaining 3 tablespoons of lemon juice and a few drops of Tabasco, cover, and place in the refrigerator to chill for 30 minutes.

6. When you're ready to eat, season the chilled soup with salt and pepper to taste and divide it among four large bowls.

7. Top the soup with the bell pepper and red onion slices, the shrimp, and the remaining cilantro, and serve.

Shrimp Soup with Cucumber and Cilantro

MAKES 3 SERVINGS
Preparation time: 15 minutes
Cooking time: 12 minutes

2 low-sodium chicken bouillon cubes
1 cucumber, peeled and thinly sliced
2 onions, thinly sliced
12 large shrimp, shelled, with tails attached
3 sprigs of fresh parsley, very finely chopped
2 sprigs of fresh cilantro, very finely chopped
1 small fresh chili, very finely chopped

1. In a large pot, bring 5 cups of water to a boil. Add the bouillon cubes and stir until dissolved.
2. Add the cucumber, onions, and shrimp, bring back to a boil, and cook for 2 minutes.
3. Remove the soup from the heat and garnish with the parsley, cilantro, and chili. Serve hot.

Chilled Cucumber Soup

MAKES 1 SERVING

Preparation time: 10 minutes, plus 1 hour for refrigeration
Cooking time: No cooking required

½ cucumber, peeled
1 garlic clove
Salt and freshly ground black pepper
1 tablespoon tomato purée
A few drops of Tabasco sauce
1 tablespoon fat-free plain Greek-style yogurt
¼ cup ice cubes

1. In a blender, process the cucumber and garlic until smooth, about 30 seconds. Season with salt and pepper to taste.

2. Add the tomato purée, Tabasco, yogurt, and ice cubes, and process until combined.

3. Pour the soup into a medium container, cover, and refrigerate for at least 1 hour. Serve chilled.

Sorrel, Spinach, and Leek Soup

MAKES 4 SERVINGS
Preparation time: 35 minutes
Cooking time: 30 minutes

2 eggs
⅛ teaspoon vegetable oil
1 onion, chopped
2 leeks (white parts only), thinly sliced
5 to 6 lettuce leaves, chopped
1 bunch of sorrel, chopped (see Note)
3 cups chopped spinach
Salt and freshly ground black pepper
2 low-sodium chicken bouillon cubes
3 fresh chives, finely chopped
1 sprig of fresh chervil, finely chopped

1. Place the eggs in a large pot and cover with cold water. Bring to a boil. Once the water is boiling, reduce the heat to a simmer and cook the eggs for 10 minutes.

2. Remove the eggs from the hot water and let them cool by running cold water over them.

3. Peel the eggs and chop them fine.

4. Heat a deep medium frying pan over medium heat. Add the oil and wipe out any excess with a paper towel.

5. Add the onion and leeks and cook until softened, stirring often, about 5 minutes.

6. Add the lettuce, sorrel, and spinach and cook, stirring often, until just wilted, about 3 minutes.

7. Add 4 cups of hot water, season with salt and pepper to taste, and add the bouillon cubes.

8. Continue cooking for 10 minutes over medium heat.
9. In a blender, process the soup until smooth, about 30 seconds.
10. Serve hot, garnished with the chopped eggs, chives, and chervil.

Note: As a substitute for sorrel, you may use the same amount of spinach, with the addition of 1 teaspoon of lemon juice.

Carrot, Fennel, and Thyme Soup

MAKES 3 SERVINGS
Preparation time: 20 minutes
Cooking time: 25 minutes

⅛ teaspoon vegetable oil
1 medium onion, diced
1 cup thinly sliced leeks (white parts only)
2 garlic cloves, very finely chopped
¼ teaspoon fennel seeds
½ teaspoon dried thyme
4 medium carrots, diced
1 fennel bulb, diced (save tops to garnish)
3½ cups low-sodium chicken stock
Salt and freshly ground black pepper

1. Place a high-sided frying pan over medium heat. Add the oil and wipe out any excess with a paper towel.
2. Add the onion, leeks, garlic, fennel seeds, and thyme. Cook, stirring constantly, until the mixture smells aromatic.
3. Add the carrots and fennel and cook for a few more minutes.
4. Add the stock, and season with salt and pepper to taste.
5. Cook over medium heat until the carrots and fennel are soft, about 5 to 7 minutes.
6. If the stock reduces noticeably, add some water.
7. Serve the soup hot, garnished with chopped fennel tops.

Cream of Zucchini Soup

MAKES 2 SERVINGS
Preparation time: 10 minutes
Cooking time: 15 minutes

1 low-sodium chicken bouillon cube
3 medium zucchini, grated
2 tablespoons fat-free ricotta
Salt and freshly ground black pepper

1. In a medium pot, bring 1½ cups of water to a boil. Add the bouillon cube and stir until it is dissolved.
2. Add the zucchini, cover, and simmer for 10 minutes, stirring often.
3. Remove the pot from the heat and add the ricotta. Season with salt and pepper to taste.
4. In a blender, process the soup until smooth, about 30 seconds. Serve hot.

Chilled Cream of Zucchini Soup

MAKES 2 SERVINGS
Preparation time: 7 minutes, plus 1 hour for chilling
Cooking time: 15 minutes

2 medium zucchini, sliced
Salt and freshly ground black pepper
2 low-sodium chicken bouillon cubes
1 cup fat-free plain Greek-style yogurt
Approximately ¼ cup ice cubes
6 fresh basil leaves, chopped

1. Place the zucchini in a small pot, cover with water, and season with salt to taste.
2. Bring the mixture to a boil, reduce the heat, and simmer for 8 minutes.

3. In the meantime, place 1 cup of water and the bouillon cubes in a separate pot. Bring the mixture to a boil and stir until the bouillon cubes are dissolved.

4. Remove the pot from the heat.

5. Drain and rinse the zucchini and transfer to a blender.

6. Add chicken broth and 1½ cups of ice water. Process until smooth, about 30 seconds.

7. Add the yogurt, and season with salt and pepper to taste.

8. Pour the soup into a medium container, cover, and refrigerate until chilled, about 1 hour.

9. To serve, ladle the chilled soup into 2 bowls. Add a couple of ice cubes to each bowl, and garnish with the chopped basil.

Greek-Style Lemon Soup

MAKES 2 SERVINGS
Preparation time: 10 minutes
Cooking time: 20 minutes

2 low-sodium chicken bouillon cubes
A pinch of saffron
2 carrots, grated
2 zucchini, grated
1 egg yolk
Grated zest and juice of 1 lemon

1. In a medium pot, bring 4¼ cups of water, the bouillon cubes, and the saffron to a boil and stir until the bouillon cubes are dissolved.

2. Add the carrots to the broth and boil for 5 minutes.

3. Add the zucchini and boil for 3 minutes.

4. Add the egg yolk, lemon zest, and lemon juice and continue cooking over low heat for 5 more minutes. Do not allow the soup to boil. Serve hot.

Quick Gazpacho

MAKES 2 SERVINGS

Preparation time: 15 minutes, plus 1 hour for chilling

Cooking time: 10 minutes

4 tomatoes, stems removed

1 red bell pepper

1 green bell pepper

2 cucumbers, peeled, seeds removed, and chopped

6 fresh mint leaves

Salt and freshly ground black pepper

1. Fill a medium pot with water and bring to a boil. Add the tomatoes and poach for 30 seconds. Remove the tomatoes from the pot, peel off the skin, and remove the seeds.
2. Turn the oven on to Broil and cook the whole bell peppers, turning every few minutes, until they are charred on all sides, about 10 minutes.
3. Immediately place the peppers in a bowl and cover it with a plate to steam.
4. Once the peppers are cool, peel off the skin and remove the seeds, then cut the peppers into chunks.
5. In a blender, process the tomatoes, peppers, cucumber, and mint until smooth, about 30 seconds. Season with salt and pepper to taste.
6. Place the soup in a medium container, cover, and refrigerate until chilled, about 1 hour. Serve chilled.

Spring Gazpacho

MAKES 4 SERVINGS

Preparation time: 20 minutes, plus 1 hour for chilling
Cooking time: No cooking required

2¼ pounds tomatoes, stems and seeds removed,
    cut into quarters
3 sprigs of fresh parsley
1 sprig of fresh basil
1 onion, quartered
1 garlic clove, chopped
1 sprig of fresh thyme, leaves removed from stem
1 sprig of fresh savory or oregano, leaves removed from stem
Salt and freshly ground black pepper

1. In a blender, process the tomatoes, parsley, basil, onion, and garlic until smooth, about 45 seconds.
2. Stir the thyme and savory leaves into the tomato mixture. Season with salt and pepper to taste.
3. Place the soup in a medium container, cover, and refrigerate until chilled, about 1 hour. Serve chilled.

Spicy Tomato Soup

MAKES 2 SERVINGS

Preparation time: 15 minutes, plus 1 hour for chilling
Cooking time: No cooking required

1 lemon
1¼ pounds tomatoes, stems and cores removed,
    roughly chopped
3 medium carrots, roughly chopped
1 stalk of celery, including the leaves, roughly chopped
Salt and freshly ground black pepper
A few drops of Tabasco sauce

1. Wash the lemon, cut it in half, and peel one half. Discard the peel, then cut the lemon (including the half with the peel remaining) into small cubes.
2. In a blender, process the tomatoes, carrots, celery, and lemon until smooth, about 30 seconds.
3. Season with salt pepper to taste, and add the Tabasco sauce.
4. Pour into a medium-size container, cover, and place in the refrigerator until chilled, about 1 hour. Serve chilled.

Fennel Soup

MAKES 3 SERVINGS
Preparation time: 20 minutes
Cooking time: 1 hour

3 fennel bulbs, thinly sliced
4¼ cups low-sodium chicken stock
4 ripe tomatoes, stems removed
3 shallots
2 garlic cloves
A few sprigs of fresh thyme
1 small dried bay leaf
Salt and freshly ground black pepper
¼ cup fat-free plain Greek-style yogurt
A few sprigs of fresh parsley, chopped

1. In a large pot, bring 2¼ cups of water, the fennel, and the stock to a boil.
2. Reduce the heat, cover, and simmer for 20 minutes.
3. While the fennel is cooking, fill a medium pot with water and bring to a boil. Add the tomatoes and poach for 30 seconds. Remove the tomatoes from the pot, peel off the skin, and remove the seeds.
4. Place the tomatoes in a food processor with the shallots and garlic cloves. Process until thoroughly combined, about 1 minute.

5. Add the tomato mixture to the fennel in the large pot. Season with the thyme and bay leaf, along with salt and pepper to taste. Continue cooking for 30 minutes. Remove the thyme and bay leaf.
6. Serve hot, garnished with the yogurt and parsley.

Chicken and Mushroom Soup

MAKES 4 SERVINGS
Preparation time: 20 minutes
Cooking time: 15 minutes

1 garlic clove
1 tablespoon fresh cilantro leaves
1 teaspoon black peppercorns
⅛ teaspoon vegetable oil
3 button mushrooms, thinly sliced
4¼ cups low-sodium chicken stock
2 tablespoons nuoc mam (Vietnamese fish sauce)
9 ounces cooked boneless, skinless chicken breast,
    cut into thin slices
2 shallots, finely chopped

1. Crush the garlic, cilantro, and peppercorns with a mortar and pestle until puréed.
2. Heat a small nonstick frying pan over medium heat. Add the oil and wipe out any excess with a paper towel.
3. Add the mushrooms and cook for 1 minute, remove them from the pan, and set aside.
4. In a medium pot, bring the stock to a boil. Add the mushrooms, nuoc mam, and garlic purée.
5. Cover, reduce the heat, and simmer for 5 minutes.
6. Add the chicken to the soup, and simmer for a few minutes to warm the chicken through. Serve hot, garnished with the chopped shallots.

Chicory and Smoked Chicken Soup

MAKES 4 SERVINGS

Preparation time: 15 minutes

Cooking time: 20 minutes

1¾ pounds chicory, chopped

4¼ cups low-sodium chicken stock

1 onion, chopped

3½ ounces smoked chicken, cut into small pieces

1. In a large pot, bring the chicory and stock to a boil. Reduce the heat and simmer for 10 minutes.
2. Heat a heavy-bottomed skillet over medium heat, add the onion and chicken, and cook, stirring continuously, until the onion is soft, about 5 minutes.
3. Add the chicken and onion to the stock pot and cook for an additional 3 minutes over medium heat. Serve hot.

Red Curried Eggplant Soup

MAKES 2 SERVINGS

Preparation time: 20 minutes

Cooking time: 45 minutes

1 eggplant

⅛ teaspoon vegetable oil

1 red onion, chopped

1 fresh green or red chili, very finely chopped

1 teaspoon curry powder

½ teaspoon ground cinnamon

¼ teaspoon ground cloves

Salt and freshly ground black pepper

2 medium tomatoes, stems and core removed, chopped

2½ cups low-sodium vegetable stock

1. Cut off the ends of the eggplant and cut into 1-inch-thick slices.

2. Heat a large saucepan over medium heat. Add the oil and wipe out any excess with a paper towel.

3. Add the onion and cook until brown, about 3 minutes. Add the chili, curry powder, cinnamon, and clove. Add salt and pepper to taste, and cook for another 2 minutes, stirring continuously.

4. Add the eggplant, tomatoes, and stock. Simmer for 40 minutes with the saucepan half covered.

5. In a blender, process the soup until smooth, about 30 seconds.

6. Reheat the soup before serving, adjusting the salt and pepper to taste.

Curried Turnip Soup with Crispy Ham

MAKES 2 SERVINGS

Preparation time: 20 minutes

Cooking time: 45 minutes

⅛ teaspoon vegetable oil

1 onion, roughly chopped

4 garlic cloves, thinly sliced

2¼ pounds turnips, peeled and quartered

A pinch of curry powder

3 cups low-sodium chicken stock

Salt and freshly ground black pepper

A few drops of Tabasco sauce

1½ tablespoons fresh lemon juice

1 cup fat-free plain Greek-style yogurt

2½ ounces thinly sliced extra-lean ham

2 sprigs of fresh parsley or 4 fresh chives, finely chopped

A pinch of ground nutmeg

1. Heat a large, heavy-bottomed pot over medium heat. Add the oil and wipe out any excess with a paper towel.

2. Add the onion and garlic and cook for 5 minutes, stirring often.

3. Add the turnip and cook for another 5 minutes, stirring often.

4. Add the curry powder and stock, bring to a simmer, and cook for 30 minutes.

5. In a blender, process the turnip mixture until very smooth, about 1 minute.

6. Season with salt and pepper to taste, and add the Tabasco and the lemon juice.

7. Reheat the soup again, and stir in ¾ cup of the yogurt.

8. Heat a heavy-bottomed skillet over medium heat, add the ham, and cook until crispy, about 5 minutes.

9. Remove the ham from the pan, drain it on paper towels, and crumble it with your fingers.

10. Serve the soup garnished with the remaining ¼ cup yogurt, crumbled ham, chopped parsley, and nutmeg.

Eugénie's Vegetable Soup

MAKES 4 SERVINGS
Preparation time: 15 minutes
Cooking time: 10 minutes

4 cups low-sodium chicken stock
Salt and freshly ground black pepper
1 carrot, cut into long, thin strips
8 small button mushrooms, chopped
1 stalk of celery, cut into long, thin strips
1 leek (white parts only), cut into long, thin strips
2 medium tomatoes, stems and seeds removed, chopped
1 bunch of fresh parsley, very finely chopped

1. In a large pot, bring the stock to a boil and season with salt and pepper to taste.

2. Add the carrot, mushrooms, celery, and leeks, and cook uncovered for 5 minutes.

3. Remove the pot from the heat and add the tomatoes and parsley. Serve hot.

Poultry and Vegetables

Smoked Chicken Canapés

MAKES 20 CANAPES

Preparation time: 45 minutes

Cooking time: 40 minutes

7 egg whites

1 tablespoon cornstarch

¼ teaspoon vegetable oil

6 ounces smoked chicken breast, diced

7 ounces button mushrooms, chopped

2 shallots, chopped

2 tablespoons plain fat-free Greek-style yogurt

1 tablespoon chopped fresh chives

Salt and freshly ground black pepper

20 fresh chives, blanched, for tying the galettes

1. In a medium bowl, whisk together the egg whites, ¼ cup of cold water, and the cornstarch.
2. Heat a large nonstick frying pan over medium heat. Add ⅛ teaspoon of the oil and wipe out any excess with a paper towel.
3. Working in batches, drop the batter into the pan by the spoonful to produce 20 round pancakes, each about 4 inches in diameter. Cook for 3 to 5 minutes until the underside is golden and the top starts to dry. Flip and cook until the other side is golden, 2 to 3 minutes. Set on paper towels to drain, and cover to keep warm.
4. Recoat the skillet with ⅛ teaspoon vegetable oil, wiping out any excess with a paper towel. Add the chicken, mushrooms, and shallots, and cook until browned, stirring constantly, about 5 minutes.
5. Lower the heat and add the yogurt and chopped chives, along with salt and pepper to taste.

6. Top the galettes with equal amounts of filling, fold the galettes over in thirds, and tie each one with a chive.

7. Keep in a cool place and serve at room temperature.

Chicken Tikka Kebabs

MAKES 4 SERVINGS

Preparation time: 25 minutes, plus 2 hours for marinating

Cooking time: 10 minutes

1 onion, quartered

1 garlic clove

1 tablespoon peeled and grated fresh ginger

2 tablespoons fresh lemon juice

Salt and freshly ground black pepper

½ cup fat-free plain Greek-style yogurt

1½ teaspoons ground coriander

1½ teaspoons ground cumin

1 teaspoon garam masala

2 tablespoons very finely chopped fresh cilantro

1¾ pounds boneless, skinless chicken breasts, cut into ¾-inch chunks

¼ onion, sliced

1 lemon, cut in wedges

½ cucumber, sliced

1. In a blender, process the quartered onion and garlic until puréed, about 30 seconds.

2. Add the ginger, lemon juice, salt and pepper to taste, yogurt, coriander, cumin, garam masala, and cilantro. Process until combined, about 10 seconds.

3. Coat the chicken with the spice mix, cover, and refrigerate for 2 hours.

4. Preheat a grill or broiler for 5 minutes.

5. Thread the chicken chunks onto skewers (see Note) and grill or broil for 5 minutes on each side.

6. Serve the kebabs hot with the sliced onion, lemon wedges, and cucumber.

Note: You will need wooden or metal skewers for this recipe. If you are using wooden skewers, soak them in water for at least 30 minutes so they won't burn.

Chicken with Mushrooms and Asparagus

MAKES 4 SERVINGS

Preparation time: 20 minutes

Cooking time: 25 minutes

⅛ teaspoon vegetable oil

2¼ pounds button mushrooms, thinly sliced

2 onions, very thinly sliced

2¼ pounds boneless, skinless chicken breasts, cut into cubes

1 pound 2 ounces asparagus tips, cut into small pieces

Juice of 1 lemon

¼ cup chopped fresh parsley

Salt and freshly ground black pepper

1. Heat a nonstick frying pan over medium heat. Add the oil and wipe out any excess with a paper towel.
2. Add the mushrooms, cook for 5 minutes, stirring often, remove from pan, and set aside.
3. Add the onion and cook until brown, about 5 minutes.
4. Add the chicken and cook until brown, about 6 minutes.
5. Add the asparagus, cooked mushrooms, lemon juice, and parsley, along with salt and pepper to taste.
6. Reduce the heat, cover, and continue cooking for 10 minutes.

Chicken Fricassee

MAKES 4 SERVINGS

Preparation time: 20 minutes

Cooking time: 1 hour

2¼ pounds skinless chicken pieces

Salt and freshly ground black pepper

⅛ teaspoon vegetable oil

9 ounces button mushrooms, thinly sliced

4 tomatoes, stems and seeds removed, quartered

2 egg yolks

1 cup fat-free plain Greek-style yogurt

1. Season the chicken with salt and pepper to taste.
2. Heat a large, heavy-bottomed pan over medium heat. Add the oil and wipe out any excess with a paper towel.
3. Add the chicken to the pan and cook until browned on all sides, about 10 minutes.
4. Add the mushrooms and ½ cup of water, reduce the heat, cover, and cook for 30 minutes.
5. Add the tomatoes and cook for an additional 10 minutes.
6. Place the egg yolks in a medium-size heat-safe bowl, add the yogurt, and mix until thoroughly combined.
7. Add ½ cup of the chicken cooking liquid to the yogurt mixture, and mix until thoroughly combined.
8. Fill a medium pot with water and bring to a simmer.
9. Place the bowl with the yogurt sauce over the pot. The bottom of the bowl should not touch the water. Heat the sauce, stirring continuously.
10. Serve the chicken with the yogurt sauce on top.

Oven-Baked Chicken Parcels with Zucchini

MAKES 4 SERVINGS

Preparation time: 10 minutes

Cooking time: 20 minutes

2 tomatoes, stems removed

⅛ teaspoon vegetable oil

4 zucchini, cut into strips

1 garlic clove, chopped

1 lemon, thinly sliced

8 boneless, skinless chicken breast cutlets, cut into tiny strips

1. Preheat oven to 425°F.
2. Cut four 8 × 10-inch rectangles of parchment paper.
3. Poach the tomatoes in boiling water for 30 seconds, then peel off the skin. Coarsely chop the poached tomatoes.
4. Heat a frying pan over medium heat. Add the oil and wipe out any excess with a paper towel.
5. Add the zucchini, tomatoes, garlic, and lemon, and cook for 5 minutes, stirring often.
6. Divide the vegetable mixture among the four pieces of parchment paper and top with equal amounts of the chicken. Fold each piece of parchment paper into a parcel and seal it with butcher's twine.
7. Place the parcels on a baking sheet and bake for 15 minutes.

Chicken with Lemon and Ginger Sauce

MAKES 4 SERVINGS

Preparation time: 30 minutes

Cooking time: 1 hour 10 minutes

1 whole chicken, about 3 pounds

1 bouquet garni (make your own by tying together 6 sprigs of fresh parsley, 3 sprigs of fresh thyme, and 3 dried bay leaves)

1 teaspoon herbes de Provence (a mix of dried marjoram, thyme, savory, basil, rosemary, sage, and fennel seeds)

1 low-sodium chicken bouillon cube

1 red bell pepper, seeds removed and cut into thin strips

Salt and freshly ground black pepper

6 carrots, sliced into 1-inch-thick pieces

1 tablespoon cornstarch

⅛ teaspoon vegetable oil

1 onion, thinly sliced

A pinch of curry powder

1 lemon, cut into quarters

1 teaspoon peeled and very thinly sliced fresh ginger

1. Fill a large casserole three-quarters full with water. Add the chicken, bouquet garni, herbes de Provence, bouillon, and red pepper, along with salt and pepper to taste.
2. Bring to a boil, reduce the heat, cover, and simmer for 50 minutes.
3. Add the carrots and continue cooking for 10 minutes.
4. In a small bowl, combine the cornstarch with 3 tablespoons of cold water and mix until smooth.
5. Heat a large nonstick frying pan over medium heat. Add the oil and wipe out any excess with a paper towel.
6. To make the sauce, add the onion, curry powder, cornstarch mixture, lemon, and ginger and cook for 5 minutes, stirring constantly, taking care not to let the sauce boil.
7. Remove the chicken from the casserole. Drain the cooking liquid but reserve the carrots.

8. Remove the skin from the chicken and discard, then cut the chicken into pieces.

9. Add the chicken pieces to the sauce, and add salt and pepper to taste. Serve with the carrots on the side.

Chicken with Chanterelle Mushrooms

MAKES 4 TO 6 SERVINGS
Preparation time: 20 minutes
Cooking time: 40 minutes

¼ teaspoon vegetable oil

6 chicken legs with thighs attached, skin removed

Salt and freshly ground black pepper

½ cup low-sodium chicken stock

1 sprig of fresh tarragon

2¼ pounds chanterelle mushrooms, cleaned and sliced

1 garlic clove, very finely chopped

1 bunch of fresh parsley, very finely chopped

1 cup fat-free plain Greek-style yogurt

1. Heat a large, heavy-bottomed skillet over medium heat. Add ⅛ teaspoon of the oil and wipe out any excess with a paper towel.

2. Season the chicken legs with salt and pepper to taste, and add them to the hot skillet. Cook until browned on both sides, about 3 minutes on each side.

3. Add the stock and tarragon, bring to a boil, lower the heat, cover, and simmer for 25 minutes.

4. Heat a nonstick frying pan over medium heat. Add the remaining ⅛ teaspoon of the oil and wipe out any excess with a paper towel. Add the mushrooms, garlic, and parsley, along with salt and pepper to taste.

5. Cook, stirring often, until the mushrooms are tender, about 5 minutes.

6. Remove the chicken and tarragon from the skillet and deglaze the pan with the yogurt, taking care not to boil the sauce. Add salt and pepper to taste.
7. Serve the chicken hot with the yogurt sauce and the mushrooms.

Note: You may substitute oyster mushrooms for the chanterelles.

Roast Herbed Chicken

MAKES 4 SERVINGS
Preparation time: 15 minutes, plus overnight refrigeration
Cooking time: 1 hour

1 bunch of fresh basil
3 garlic cloves, chopped
1 lemon, cut into quarters
3 sprigs of fresh thyme
3 sprigs of fresh rosemary
1 whole chicken, about 3 pounds
1 cup leeks, white parts only, finely chopped
4 carrots, finely chopped
Salt and freshly ground black pepper

1. In a small mixing bowl, combine the basil, garlic, lemon, thyme, and rosemary and stuff the mixture inside the chicken.
2. Wrap the chicken and refrigerate overnight.
3. The following day, preheat oven to 425°F.
4. Place the leeks and carrots in a deep roasting pan, season with salt and pepper to taste, and add ½ cup of water.
5. Place the chicken atop the vegetables and roast until a thermometer inserted into the middle of the chicken registers 170°F, or until the juices run clear when a knife is pierced into the thickest part of the thigh, about 1 hour.
6. Remove the skin from the chicken before serving.
7. Serve hot, garnished with the leeks and carrots.

Chicken with Mushrooms

MAKES 4 SERVINGS
Preparation time: 20 minutes
Cooking time: 35 minutes

1¼ pounds button mushrooms, ends removed and thinly sliced,
    tops whole
1 tablespoon fresh lemon juice
Salt and freshly ground black pepper
1 onion, chopped
1 pound 12 ounces boneless, skinless chicken breasts,
    cut into cubes
2 tomatoes, stems and seeds removed, chopped
2 garlic cloves, chopped
1 cup low-sodium chicken stock

1. In a medium bowl, toss the mushrooms with the lemon juice. Add salt and pepper to taste and place in a large nonstick, heatproof casserole.
2. Cover and cook over low heat until all the liquid has evaporated.
3. Remove the mushrooms from the casserole and set them aside.
4. Place the onion and 2 tablespoons of water in the casserole and cook until browned.
5. Add the chicken, tomatoes, cooked mushrooms, garlic, and chicken stock, plus salt and pepper to taste.
6. Bring to a simmer, cover, and cook over low heat for 20 minutes.

Stir-Fried Chicken with Peppers and Bamboo Shoots

MAKES 4 SERVINGS

Preparation time: 15 minutes, plus 2 hours for marinating

Cooking time: 20 minutes

4 boneless, skinless chicken breasts, cut into strips

2 tablespoons low-sodium soy sauce

2 teaspoons peeled and grated fresh ginger

1 garlic clove, thinly sliced

2 sprigs of fresh mint, leaves removed (and stems discarded), very finely chopped

2 sprigs of fresh cilantro, leaves removed (and stems discarded), very finely chopped

1 green bell pepper

1 red bell pepper

⅛ teaspoon vegetable oil

1 onion, thinly sliced

5 ounces canned bamboo shoots, rinsed and chopped

Salt and freshly ground black pepper

1. Place the chicken strips in a shallow nonreactive dish and add the soy sauce, ginger, garlic, mint, and cilantro.
2. Cover and marinate in the refrigerator for 2 hours.
3. While the chicken is marinating, turn the oven to Broil and roast the peppers until charred all over, about 5 minutes on each side.
4. Immediately place the peppers in a bowl and place a plate on top to steam. Once the peppers have cooled, peel off the skin, remove the seeds, and cut the peppers into strips.
5. After the chicken has marinated, drain and strain the marinade into a small bowl, discarding the solids that don't fit through the strainer and reserving the liquid.
6. Heat a large nonstick frying pan over medium heat. Add the oil and wipe out any excess with a paper towel.
7. Add the chicken and cook until brown, stirring often, about 5 minutes.

8. Add the onion and cook until golden brown, then add the peppers and continue cooking for an additional 4 minutes.
9. Add the reserved marinade and cook for 3 more minutes.
10. Stir in the bamboo shoots and heat for an additional minute. Season with salt and pepper to taste before serving.

Basque Chicken

MAKES 4 SERVINGS
Preparation time: 15 minutes
Cooking time: 1 hour 5 minutes

2¼ pounds tomatoes, stems and seeds removed
1 whole chicken, about 3 pounds, cut into 8 pieces
Salt and freshly ground black pepper
⅛ teaspoon vegetable oil
1 carrot, diced
2 green bell peppers, seeds removed, diced
2 garlic cloves, chopped
1 bouquet garni (make your own by tying together 6 sprigs of fresh parsley, 3 sprigs of fresh thyme, and 3 dried bay leaves)

1. Poach the tomatoes in boiling water for 30 seconds, then peel off the skin and remove the seeds.
2. Season the chicken with salt and pepper to taste.
3. Heat a large nonstick skillet over medium heat. Add the oil and wipe out any excess with a paper towel.
4. Add the chicken and cook until browned on all sides, about 5 minutes.
5. Add the tomatoes, carrot, bell peppers, garlic, and bouquet garni, along with salt and pepper to taste.
6. Reduce the heat, cover, and simmer for 1 hour.
7. Remove the skin from the chicken before serving.

Chicken Marengo

MAKES 4 SERVINGS

Preparation time: 30 minutes

Cooking time: 1 hour

⅛ teaspoon vegetable oil

1 whole chicken, about 3 pounds, cut into 8 pieces

2 onions, sliced

2 shallots, sliced

1 garlic clove, sliced

2 tablespoons white wine vinegar

1 tablespoon tomato purée

4 tomatoes, stems and seeds removed, diced

Salt and freshly ground black pepper

3 sprigs of fresh thyme

1 dried bay leaf

3 sprigs of fresh parsley

1. Heat a large heavy-bottomed nonstick skillet over medium heat. Add the oil and wipe out any excess with a paper towel.
2. Add the chicken and cook until browned on all sides, about 5 minutes.
3. Remove the chicken from the skillet and add the onions, shallots, and garlic. Cook, stirring often, for 2 minutes.
4. Add 1 cup of water and the vinegar, tomato purée, and tomatoes.
5. Transfer the chicken pieces back to the skillet and season with salt and pepper to taste.
6. Add the thyme, bay leaf, and parsley, reduce the heat, cover, and simmer for 45 minutes. Remove the bay leaf.
7. Remove the skin from the chicken before serving.

Poached Chicken in a Light Herb Sauce

MAKES 4 SERVINGS

Preparation time: 30 minutes

Cooking time: 1 hour

½ lemon

1 whole chicken, about 3 pounds

1 onion, cut in half, each half studded with a clove

1 carrot, quartered

2 whole leeks, tied together

1 celery stick

1 bouquet garni (make your own by tying together 6 sprigs
of fresh parsley, 3 sprigs of fresh thyme, and 3 dried bay
leaves)

1 garlic clove, cut in half

Salt

FOR THE SAUCE

2 egg yolks

2 tablespoons fat-free plain Greek-style yogurt

1 teaspoon chopped fresh herbs, singly or mixed, such as
chives, tarragon, parsley, and chervil

1. Rub the lemon half over the surface of the chicken, then
place the chicken in a large casserole.

2. Add the onion, carrot, leeks, celery, bouquet garni, and
garlic.

3. Fill the casserole with cold water to ¾ inch above the chicken,
then add a pinch of salt to taste.

4. Place the casserole on the stove over high heat and bring the
liquid to a boil. Skim off any foam with a ladle, reduce the
heat, and simmer for 40 minutes.

5. Drain the chicken over a bowl, and set aside ⅔ cup of the
chicken stock. Skim off any fat and keep the stock warm.

6. To make the sauce, put the egg yolks in a heatproof bowl and
add 1 tablespoon of cold water.

7. Bring a pan of water to a simmer and place the bowl over the pan, making sure the bottom of the bowl does not touch the water.

8. Beat the eggs until creamy, taking care not to overheat them.

9. Whisk in the yogurt, then add the reserved warm stock, stirring continuously. Add the herbs.

10. Remove the skin from the chicken and serve piping hot with the sauce.

Yogurt and Herbed Chicken Salad

MAKES 2 SERVINGS
Preparation time: 15 minutes
Cooking time: No cooking required

⅔ cup fat-free plain Greek-style yogurt
1 garlic clove, chopped
1 teaspoon mustard
3 sprigs of fresh parsley, chopped
3 fresh chives, finely chopped
Salt and freshly ground black pepper
10 ounces button mushrooms, cut into small cubes
1 bunch of radishes, greens discarded, cut into small cubes
4 slices cooked chicken with herbs, diced
4 large gherkin pickles, cut into thick slices*

1. In a large bowl, combine the yogurt, garlic, mustard, parsley, and chives, along with salt and pepper to taste.

2. Add the mushrooms, radishes, chicken, and pickles, and toss until the dressing is evenly distributed.

*Use only no-sugar-added pickles.

Chicken Provençal

MAKES 4 SERVINGS

Preparation time: 15 minutes

Cooking time: 1 hour

⅛ teaspoon vegetable oil

1 whole chicken, about 3 pounds, cut into 8 pieces

1 (15-ounce) can of diced tomatoes

4 garlic cloves, crushed

1 small bunch of fresh parsley, finely chopped

Salt and freshly ground black pepper

1. Heat a large nonstick skillet over medium heat. Add the oil and wipe out any excess with a paper towel.
2. Add the chicken and cook until browned on all sides, about 5 minutes, then remove from pan and set aside.
3. Add the chopped tomatoes, garlic, and parsley to the skillet, along with salt and pepper to taste.
4. Reduce the heat, cover, and simmer for 30 minutes.
5. Return the chicken pieces to the skillet (if dry, add ½ cup of water).
6. Cover and continue cooking for 20 minutes.
7. Remove the skin from the chicken before serving.

Tarragon Chicken Terrine

MAKES 6 SERVINGS

Preparation time: 40 minutes, plus 24 hours for refrigeration

Cooking time: 1 hour 50 minutes

1 whole chicken, about 3 pounds

2¼ cups low-sodium chicken stock

2 leeks, white parts only, cleaned

3 carrots

2 garlic cloves

1 onion, cut into quarters

1 bunch of fresh tarragon

Salt and freshly ground black pepper

1 pound chicken livers

1½ (7-gram) envelopes (10½ grams or 1 tablespoon total) of unflavored gelatin

1. Place the chicken in a large casserole, pour in the stock, and add cold water until the chicken is completely submerged.
2. Add the leeks, carrots, garlic, onion, and half the tarragon, along with salt and pepper to taste.
3. Place the casserole on the stove and bring the liquid to a boil over high heat.
4. Reduce the heat, cover, and cook for 45 minutes, skimming the fat off the top at regular intervals.
5. Add the chicken livers and continue cooking for an additional 45 minutes.
6. With a slotted spoon, remove the chicken, chicken livers, carrots, and leeks from the casserole. Dice them all into large cubes and set aside separately.
7. Heat the stock over medium heat and simmer until reduced by half, then strain into a medium bowl.
8. Add the gelatin to the stock and mix until thoroughly dissolved.
9. Line the bottom of a 9-inch loaf pan with the remaining tarragon and pour in a little of the stock.

10. In the loaf pan, layer the diced ingredients, starting with half of the herbed chicken, half the chicken livers, half the carrots, and half the leeks. Repeat.

11. Pour the stock over the top, cover, and refrigerate for 24 hours.

Note: You will need a 9-inch loaf pan for this recipe. Prepare this recipe the day before you wish to serve it.

Chicken and Pepper Kebabs

MAKES 4 SERVINGS

Preparation time: 30 minutes, plus overnight marinating

Cooking time: 10 minutes

4 boneless, skinless chicken breasts, cut into ¾-inch cubes

4 garlic cloves, chopped

¼ cup fresh lemon juice

1 teaspoon ground cumin

1 teaspoon dried thyme

Salt and freshly ground black pepper

1 green or red bell pepper, seeds removed, cut into cubes

8 shallots, quartered

1. Place the chicken in a shallow dish and toss with the garlic, lemon juice, cumin, and thyme. Add salt and pepper to taste.
2. Cover and refrigerate overnight.
3. The next day, preheat the oven to Broil (or a grill to High).
4. Thread the chicken pieces onto skewers (see Note), alternating chicken, bell pepper, and shallots.
5. Brush the kebabs with the marinade and cook under the broiler or on the barbecue, 5 minutes on each side.

Note: You will need wooden or metal skewers for this recipe. If you are using wooden skewers, soak them in water for at least 30 minutes so they won't burn.

Herbed Chicken Roulade

MAKES 2 SERVINGS
Preparation time: 15 minutes
Cooking time: 20 minutes

1 egg
¼ cup chopped radishes
2 shallots, chopped
¼ cup peeled and chopped cucumber
3 to 4 fresh chives, chopped
3 sprigs of fresh parsley, chopped
A pinch of chopped fresh tarragon
1 cup fat-free plain Greek-style yogurt
Salt and freshly ground black pepper
4 slices of cooked chicken
1 tomato, stem removed, cut in half
4 small gherkin pickles*

1. Place the egg in a small pot and cover with cold water. Bring to a boil. Once the water is boiling, reduce the heat to a simmer and cook the egg for 10 minutes.
2. Remove the egg from the hot water and let it cool by running it under cold water. Peel the egg and cut it in half.
3. In a medium bowl, mix the radishes with the shallots, cucumber, chives, parsley, tarragon, and yogurt. Add salt and pepper to taste.
4. Spread this mixture over the 4 chicken slices and roll up each slice, securing each roll with a toothpick.
5. To serve, place 2 of the rolls on each of 2 plates, along with half a tomato, half a hard-boiled egg, and a couple of gherkins.

*Use only no-sugar-added pickles.

Summer Terrine

MAKES 4 TO 6 SERVINGS

Preparation time: 30 minutes, plus 4 hours for cooling and refrigeration

Cooking time: 1 hour 20 minutes

2¼ cups low-sodium vegetable or chicken stock

2¼ pounds green beans

1 carrot

1 stick of celery

1 onion

5 sprigs of fresh tarragon, chopped

½ teaspoon chopped fresh oregano

8 slices of extra-lean ham (or cooked turkey or chicken)

4 eggs

⅔ cup fat-free plain Greek-style yogurt

1 tablespoon fat-free cream cheese (optional)

Salt and freshly ground black pepper

1. Preheat oven to 350°F.
2. Line an 8-cup loaf pan with parchment paper, allowing the paper to overlap the longest sides of the pan.
3. In a medium-size pot, bring the stock to a boil, add the green beans, and cook for 3 minutes.
4. Drain the beans, then cut them into small pieces.
5. In a food processor or blender, process the carrot, celery, and onion until roughly chopped.
6. Heat a large nonstick frying pan over medium heat.
7. Add the carrot mixture to the pan and cook for 10 minutes, stirring often.
8. Add the beans to the pan and cook, stirring often, until the beans no longer drain off any water, about 5 minutes.
9. Add the tarragon and oregano.
10. Line the loaf pan with 6 slices of the ham, allowing the slices to spill over the sides, and top with the vegetable mixture.
11. In a medium bowl, beat together the eggs, yogurt, and cream cheese (if using). Add salt and pepper to taste.

12. Pour the egg mixture over the vegetable mixture.

13. Fold the ends of the ham over the egg mixture and cover with the remaining 2 slices of ham.

14. Cover the top of the pan with aluminum foil and place it in a larger baking dish. Fill this larger dish halfway with cold water.

15. Place the baking dish in the oven and bake the terrine for 1 hour.

16. Remove the loaf pan from the baking dish and allow to cool for about 20 minutes.

17. Cover and refrigerate for 4 hours before serving.

Note: You will need an 8-cup loaf pan for this recipe.

Roast Lemon Cornish Hen with Cherry Tomatoes

MAKES 2 SERVINGS
Preparation time: 20 minutes
Cooking time: 30 minutes

2 Cornish hens
1 tablespoon fresh thyme
1 lemon, cut into slices
2¼ cups low-sodium chicken stock
2 medium onions, thinly sliced
1 pound 9 ounces cherry tomatoes
2 garlic cloves, chopped
Salt and freshly ground black pepper

1. Preheat oven to 350°F.

2. Place the Cornish hens in a deep baking dish and top with the thyme and lemon slices.

3. Place in the oven and bake for 10 minutes, then remove from the oven.

4. Add the chicken stock and arrange the onions, tomatoes, and garlic around the hen.

5. Season with salt and pepper to taste, and stir the cooking juices so that the tomatoes are coated with them.
6. Cook for an additional 20 minutes.
7. Remove the skin from the hens before serving.

Turkey Drumsticks with Red Bell Peppers

MAKES 2 SERVINGS
Preparation time: 30 minutes
Cooking time: 1 hour

2 turkey drumsticks
3 red bell peppers
2 tablespoons red wine vinegar
2 tablespoons fat-free plain Greek-style yogurt
Salt and freshly ground black pepper

1. Heat a heavy-bottomed skillet over medium heat.
2. Add the drumsticks and 2 tablespoons of water and cook until the turkey is browned, about 5 minutes on each side.
3. Reduce the heat, cover, and cook the drumsticks for 40 minutes, turning them every 10 minutes.
4. Turn oven on to Broil and cook the bell peppers, turning every few minutes, until they are charred on all sides, about 10 minutes.
5. Immediately place the peppers in a bowl and put a plate on top.
6. Once the peppers have cooled, peel off the skin, remove the seeds, then cut the peppers into chunks.
7. In a blender, process the peppers until puréed.
8. Remove the drumsticks from the skillet and keep warm.
9. Deglaze the skillet with the vinegar.
10. In a small bowl, stir together the yogurt and bell pepper purée, adding salt and pepper to taste.
11. Add the yogurt sauce to the skillet and heat to a simmer. Do not let the sauce boil.

12. To serve, arrange the drumsticks on a dish, remove the skins, and cover them with the sauce.

Leek and Turkey Bake

MAKES 2 SERVINGS
Preparation time: 20 minutes
Cooking time: 35 minutes

¼ teaspoon vegetable oil
1¾ pounds leeks (white parts only), thinly sliced
7 ounces cooked turkey slices
1 shallot, very finely chopped
2 eggs
3 ounces fat-free plain Greek-style yogurt
Salt

1. Preheat oven to 375°F.
2. Add ⅛ teaspoon of the oil to a 9-inch-square baking dish, using a paper towel to coat it and to wipe out any excess.
3. Fill the bottom part of a large steamer with water and bring to a simmer.
4. Place the leeks in the top part of the steamer, cover, and steam for 10 minutes.
5. Heat a heavy-bottomed skillet over medium heat. Add the remaining oil and wipe out any excess with a paper towel.
6. Add the turkey slices and shallot and cook until brown, about 5 minutes.
7. In a medium bowl, whisk together the eggs, yogurt, and salt to taste.
8. In a separate bowl, combine the turkey mixture with the leeks.
9. Place the turkey and leek mixture in the prepared baking dish and top with the egg mixture.
10. Place the dish in the oven and bake until golden brown on top, about 20 minutes.

Note: You will need a large steamer for this recipe.

Ham and Turkey Rolls

MAKES 4 SERVINGS
Preparation time: 30 minutes
Cooking time: 50 minutes

1½ pounds boneless, skinless turkey breast
⅛ teaspoon vegetable oil
3½ ounces button mushrooms, stems removed and chopped,
    tops whole
1 onion, chopped
1 tablespoon chopped fresh parsley
Salt and freshly ground black pepper
4 slices of extra-lean ham
2¼ cups low-sodium chicken stock

1. Place the turkey breast between two sheets of plastic wrap and pound with a meat mallet or small skillet until it is ⅛ inch thick. Cut into 4 portions.
2. Heat a heavy-bottomed skillet over medium heat. Add the oil and wipe out any excess with a paper towel.
3. Add the mushroom stems, half of the chopped onion, and the parsley. Cook for 5 minutes. Remove the mixture from the pan, season with salt and pepper to taste, and reserve.
4. Place a slice of ham atop each portion of turkey, and spoon a quarter of the mushroom mixture in the center.
5. Roll each slice over the filling and tie it with a piece of butcher's twine.
6. Brown the turkey rolls in the skillet, about 3 minutes on each side, remove, and place in a casserole.
7. Add the remaining chopped onion, the stock, 1 cup of water, and salt and pepper to taste. Cover and simmer for 15 minutes.
8. Add the mushroom tops and cook for an additional 20 minutes. Remove the twine, and serve.

Chicken with Savoy Cabbage

MAKES 4 SERVINGS
Preparation time: 30 minutes
Cooking time: 1 hour

Half a lemon
1 whole chicken, about 3 pounds
Salt and freshly ground black pepper
1 head of Savoy cabbage, cut into 8 pieces
1 onion, cut in quarters, with a clove inserted in each quarter
1 bouquet garni (make your own by tying together 6 sprigs
    of fresh parsley, 3 sprigs of fresh thyme, and 3 dried bay
    leaves)
2¼ cups low-sodium chicken stock

1. Preheat oven to 425°F.
2. Rub the lemon over the chicken, place the chicken on a baking sheet, and bake for 5 minutes.
3. While the chicken is baking, fill a large pot with water, season with a pinch of salt, and bring to a boil.
4. Blanch the cabbage for 5 minutes, then drain.
5. Transfer the chicken to a heatproof casserole and surround it with the cabbage.
6. Add the onion, bouquet garni, pepper, and chicken stock.
7. Cover and bake for 50 minutes, basting the chicken regularly.
8. Once the bird is cooked, take the casserole out of the oven and drain the stock into a medium saucepan.
9. Place the saucepan over medium-high heat on top of the stove, and reduce the stock as much as possible, then season with salt and pepper to taste.
10. Remove the skin from the chicken and pour the stock over the chicken before serving.

Meat and Vegetables

Poached Filet of Beef

MAKES 1 SERVING
Preparation time: 20 minutes
Cooking time: 35 minutes

1 bouquet garni (make your own by tying together 6 sprigs of
fresh parsley, 3 sprigs of fresh thyme, and 3 dried
bay leaves)
½ onion
1 medium carrot, roughly chopped
1 leek (white part only), thinly sliced
2 stalks of celery, roughly chopped
Salt and freshly ground black pepper
9 ounces filet of beef, also known as beef chuck tender

1. In a medium pot, combine 4 cups of water, the bouquet garni, onion, carrot, leek, and celery. Add salt and pepper to taste and bring to a boil.
2. Reduce the heat, add the beef, cover, and simmer, taking care not to boil, until the beef is tender when tested with a fork, about 30 minutes.
3. Remove the meat and vegetables from the dish, slice the meat, and serve with the vegetables.

Beef with Eggplant

MAKES 4 SERVINGS

Preparation time: 20 minutes

Cooking time: 1 hour 5 minutes

⅛ teaspoon vegetable oil

10 ounces eggplant, peeled and cut into thin slices,
about ⅛ inch thick

Salt and freshly ground black pepper

3 medium tomatoes, stems removed, quartered

1 garlic clove, finely chopped

1 tablespoon fresh parsley, chopped

1 pound lean beef, such as sirloin tip or flank steak cut across
the grain into thin strips

1. Preheat oven to 425°F.
2. Add the oil to a 9 × 9-inch baking dish, using a paper towel to coat it and to wipe out any excess.
3. Sprinkle the eggplant with a little salt and place in a colander to let the juices drain, about 15 minutes.
4. In a heatproof casserole, combine the tomatoes, garlic, and parsley, and cook over medium heat, stirring often, until the edges begin to boil.
5. Reduce the heat and cook the tomatoes over low heat for 30 minutes.
6. Place half the eggplant in the prepared baking dish, and top with half of the tomatoes. Place the meat in a layer on top of the vegetables, and top with a layer of the remaining eggplant and tomatoes.
7. Bake for 30 minutes. Season with salt and pepper to taste.

Beef and Red Bell Peppers

MAKES 4 SERVINGS

Preparation time: 20 minutes, plus 2 hours for marinating

Cooking time: 50 minutes

6 tablespoons low-sodium soy sauce

1 teaspoon cornstarch

12 ounces sirloin steak, thinly sliced

⅛ teaspoon vegetable oil

2 red bell peppers, seeds removed and thinly sliced

3 small onions, quartered

Salt and freshly ground black pepper

1. In a small bowl, thoroughly combine 4 tablespoons of the soy sauce with the cornstarch.
2. Place the soy sauce marinade in a nonreactive shallow dish, add the beef, and coat it with the marinade.
3. Cover and place in the refrigerator for 2 hours to marinate.
4. When the meat has marinated, place a heavy-bottomed skillet over medium heat. Add the oil and wipe out any excess with a paper towel.
5. Add the bell peppers and onions and cook, stirring often, for 5 minutes.
6. Add 1 cup of water to the bell pepper mixture, bring it to a simmer, and cook over low heat for 30 minutes.
7. Remove the meat from the marinade and add it to the bell pepper mixture.
8. Add the 2 remaining tablespoons of soy sauce. If the sauce is very thick, add 2 tablespoons of water.
9. Cook for 15 minutes and season with salt and pepper to taste.

Beef Bourguignon

MAKES 6 SERVINGS
Preparation time: 10 minutes
Cooking time: 2 hours

¼ teaspoon vegetable oil
1 pound 2 ounces lean beef, such as sirloin tip or flank steak,
    cut into cubes
2 low-sodium beef bouillon cubes
1 teaspoon cornstarch
1 teaspoon fresh parsley, chopped
1 garlic clove, finely chopped
1 dried bay leaf
Salt and freshly ground black pepper
3 medium onions, finely chopped
5½ ounces button mushrooms, sliced

1. Preheat oven to 400°F.
2. Heat a large, heavy-bottomed skillet over medium heat. Add ⅛ teaspoon of the oil and wipe out any excess with a paper towel.
3. Add the beef and cook until browned, about 5 minutes, stirring constantly, then remove it to a casserole.
4. Add 4 cups of water to the same skillet, bring to a boil, and stir in the bouillon cubes until dissolved.
5. Add the cornstarch, parsley, garlic, and bay leaf, along with salt and pepper to taste, and whisk until the cornstarch is dissolved.
6. Bring the broth mixture to a boil, reduce the heat, and simmer, stirring often, until slightly thickened, about 15 minutes.
7. Pour the sauce over the beef, cover, and bake for 30 minutes.
8. While the beef is baking, heat a medium heavy-bottomed skillet over medium heat. Add ⅛ teaspoon of oil and wipe out any excess with a paper towel. Add the onions and mushrooms.
9. Cook, stirring often, until browned, about 7 minutes. Remove the pan from the heat and set aside.

10. After the beef has cooked for 30 minutes, add the onion and mushrooms to the casserole, cover, and continue cooking for an additional 30 minutes.

Mexican-Style Meatballs

MAKES 2 SERVINGS

Preparation time: 20 minutes

Cooking time: 25 minutes

10 ounces 95% lean ground beef

½ teaspoon Mexican spice mixture (make your own with chili powder, cumin, cayenne, paprika, and garlic powder)

Salt and freshly ground black pepper

2 medium tomatoes, stems and seeds removed

⅛ teaspoon vegetable oil

1. In a medium bowl, mix together the ground beef, ¼ teaspoon of the spice mixture, and salt and pepper to taste (the amount of salt will depend on the amount of salt in the spice mix). Mold the mixture into 4 meatballs.

2. Bring a medium pot of water to a boil, poach the tomatoes for 30 seconds, then peel off the skin, remove the seeds, and chop them fine.

3. Place the tomatoes in a medium saucepan, add the remaining ¼ teaspoon of the spice mixture, and cook over low heat until the tomatoes are soft, about 15 minutes.

4. While the tomatoes are cooking, heat a large, heavy-bottomed skillet over medium heat. Add the oil and wipe out any excess with a paper towel.

5. Add the meatballs and cook until browned on all sides, being careful not to overcook, or they will become dry, about 10 minutes.

6. To serve, pour the sauce over the meatballs.

Beef and Zucchini Ragout

MAKES 4 SERVINGS
Preparation time: 20 minutes
Cooking time: 30 minutes

2¼ pounds zucchini, sliced
⅛ teaspoon vegetable oil
1 pound 95% lean ground beef
½ cup tomato paste
1¼ cups canned crushed tomatoes
1 garlic clove, finely chopped
3 sprigs of fresh parsley, finely chopped
Salt and freshly ground black pepper

1. Fill the bottom part of a large steamer halfway with water and bring to a simmer.
2. Place the zucchini in the top part of the steamer, cover, and steam for 5 minutes. Remove the zucchini and set aside so that it doesn't overcook.
3. In the meantime, heat a large nonstick frying pan over medium heat. Add the oil and wipe out any excess with a paper towel.
4. Add the meat and cook until browned, stirring often, about 10 minutes.
5. Add the tomato paste, crushed tomatoes, garlic, parsley, and salt and pepper to taste.
6. Bring to a simmer and cook for 15 minutes.
7. When ready to serve, stir the zucchini into the meat mixture.

Note: You will need a steamer for this recipe.

Hungarian-Style Ground Beef

MAKES 3 TO 4 SERVINGS

Preparation time: 15 minutes

Cooking time: 20 minutes

⅛ teaspoon vegetable oil

6 small shallots, chopped

1 red bell pepper, seeds removed, diced

1½ pounds 95% lean ground beef

1 tablespoon paprika

½ cup tomato paste

A pinch of cayenne pepper

Salt and freshly ground black pepper

Juice of ½ lemon

⅓ cup fat-free plain Greek-style yogurt

1. Heat a heavy-bottomed skillet over medium heat. Add the oil and wipe out any excess with a paper towel.
2. Add the shallots and bell pepper and cook for 5 minutes, stirring often. Remove and set aside.
3. Add the ground beef to the hot skillet and cook for 5 minutes, crushing the meat with a fork until crumbled.
4. Add the paprika, tomato paste, and shallots and bell pepper mixture.
5. Cook for an additional 5 minutes, stirring well. Season with the cayenne and salt and pepper to taste.
6. In a small bowl, whisk the lemon juice and yogurt until thoroughly combined.
7. Remove the skillet from the heat, and stir in the yogurt mixture.
8. Return the skillet to the stove and warm the beef over low heat, without allowing the sauce to boil. Serve warm.

Sautéed Beef with Vegetables

MAKES 4 SERVINGS

Preparation time: 30 minutes, plus 30 minutes for marinating

Cooking time: 10 minutes

6 tablespoons low-sodium soy sauce

1 tablespoon sherry vinegar

1 tablespoon cornstarch

1 pound beef tenderloin, trimmed of all fat and
    thinly sliced

⅛ teaspoon vegetable oil

1 bunch of scallions, thinly sliced lengthwise

1 green bell pepper, seeds removed, cut into thin strips

2 carrots, cut into medium slices

1 teaspoon zero-calorie sweetener suited for cooking and
    baking, such as Splenda

Salt and freshly ground black pepper

1. In a shallow dish, combine the soy sauce, sherry vinegar, and cornstarch, and mix until thoroughly combined. Add the beef and cover with the marinade.
2. Cover and refrigerate for 30 minutes.
3. Remove the meat from the marinade and set both aside.
4. Heat a large, heavy-bottomed skillet over high heat. Add the oil and wipe out any excess with a paper towel.
5. Place the meat in the skillet and cook until browned, stirring continuously, about 3 minutes. Remove the meat and cover to keep warm.
6. Add the scallions, green pepper, and carrots to the hot pan and cook, stirring constantly, for 3 minutes.
7. Add the marinade, beef, and sweetener, plus salt and pepper to taste. Mix until thoroughly combined. Heat, stirring constantly, for about 2 minutes. Serve warm.

Turgloff Beef Kebabs

MAKES 2 SERVINGS
Preparation time: 20 minutes
Cooking time: 25 minutes

1 pound tomatoes, stems and seeds removed, chopped
1 garlic clove, crushed
Salt and freshly ground black pepper
1¼ pounds lean beef, such as sirloin tip or flank steak,
    cut into cubes
2 medium green bell peppers, seeds removed, cut into cubes
2 medium onions, cut into cubes
Juice of 1 lemon
A pinch of celery salt
¼ cup chopped fresh parsley

1. Preheat a grill or broiler to High.
2. Fill a medium pot with water and bring to a boil. Poach the tomatoes for 30 seconds, remove them from the water, peel off the skin, remove the seeds, and crush.
3. Place the tomatoes and garlic in a small saucepan, bring to a simmer, cook for 15 minutes, then season with salt and pepper to taste.
4. Thread the beef, bell peppers, and onions onto skewers (see Note) and grill or broil for about 5 minutes on each side.
5. To serve, remove the meat and vegetables from the skewers, divide between two plates, sprinkle with lemon juice, and season with celery salt. Serve with the tomato sauce and garnish with chopped parsley.

Note: You will need 6 wooden or metal skewers for this recipe. If you are using wooden skewers, soak them in water for at least 30 minutes before using so they won't burn.

Beef Omelet Rolls

MAKES 4 SERVINGS

Preparation time: 30 minutes, plus at least 3 hours
or overnight for marinating
Cooking time: 50 minutes

1 pound 9 ounces beef tenderloin, thinly sliced

2 tablespoons low-sodium soy sauce

2 garlic cloves, crushed

1 teaspoon peeled and grated fresh ginger

10 eggs

Salt and freshly ground black pepper

⅛ teaspoon vegetable oil

1 large onion, finely chopped

1 carrot, finely chopped

4 ounces bean sprouts

6 fresh chives, chopped

1. In a nonreactive dish, combine the beef with 1 tablespoon of the soy sauce and the garlic and ginger.
2. Cover and refrigerate for at least 3 hours, or overnight.
3. In a medium bowl, beat the eggs, ¼ cup water, and salt and pepper to taste.
4. Heat a large heavy-bottomed skillet over medium heat. Add the oil and wipe out any excess with a paper towel.
5. Make 8 thin omelets, one at a time. Cover the cooked omelets and keep them warm.
6. Add the marinated beef and onion to the hot skillet and cook, stirring often, until the meat is browned, about 5 minutes.
7. Add the remaining 1 tablespoon of soy sauce and cook until the liquid starts to boil.
8. Stir in the chopped carrot and cook for 5 minutes, then add the bean sprouts and chives. Mix until thoroughly combined.
9. To serve, place some of the beef mixture in the center of each omelet and roll up the omelet.

Meat Loaf with Mushrooms

MAKES 4 TO 6 SERVINGS
Preparation time: 20 minutes
Cooking time: 55 minutes

2 eggs, beaten
14 ounces 95% lean ground beef
14 ounces lean ground veal
1 onion, finely chopped
2 garlic cloves, crushed
Salt and freshly ground black pepper
3 sprigs of fresh thyme, finely chopped
3 sprigs of fresh rosemary, finely chopped
3 sprigs of fresh parsley, finely chopped
⅛ teaspoon vegetable oil
5 ounces button mushrooms, very finely chopped

1. Preheat oven to 475°F.
2. In a medium bowl, combine the eggs, beef, veal, onion, and garlic, plus salt and pepper to taste. Add the herbs.
3. Place a medium heavy-bottomed skillet over medium heat. Add the oil and wipe out any excess with a paper towel.
4. Add the mushrooms and cook until soft, about 7 minutes.
5. Combine the mushrooms with the meat mixture.
6. Place the mixture in a 9-inch loaf pan and bake for 45 minutes.
7. Slice, and serve hot or cold.

Note: You will need a 9-inch loaf pan for this recipe.

Cauliflower Shepherd's Pie

MAKES 6 SERVINGS
Preparation time: 20 minutes
Cooking time: 1 hour

2 pounds cauliflower, cut into florets
1¼ pounds 95% lean ground beef
1 onion, chopped
2 garlic cloves, chopped
1 small bunch of fresh parsley, chopped
Salt and freshly ground black pepper

1. Preheat oven to 350°F.
2. Fill the bottom part of a large steamer halfway with water and bring to a simmer.
3. Place the cauliflower in the top part of the steamer, cover, and steam for 10 minutes.
4. In a blender, process the cauliflower until puréed, about 1 minute.
5. In a medium bowl, combine the beef, onion, garlic, parsley, and salt and pepper to taste.
6. Place the beef mixture in a 9 × 9-inch baking dish, top with cauliflower, and bake for 45 minutes.

Note: You will need a steamer for this recipe.

Two-Pepper Beef Stew

MAKES 4 SERVINGS
Preparation time: 20 minutes
Cooking time: 40 minutes

⅛ teaspoon vegetable oil
1 pound lean beef, such as sirloin tip or flank steak, diced
½ onion, chopped
1 garlic clove, chopped
1 tablespoon tomato paste
2¼ cups low-sodium beef stock
Salt and freshly ground black pepper
1 green bell pepper, seeds removed, cut into strips
1 red bell pepper, seeds removed, cut into strips
1 carrot, chopped
1 turnip, peeled and chopped
1 tablespoon cornstarch

1. Heat a large, heavy-bottomed skillet over high heat. Add the oil and wipe out any excess with a paper towel.
2. Add the beef and cook, stirring continuously, until brown, about 5 minutes.
3. Add the onion and garlic and continue cooking for 1 minute, stirring continuously.
4. Add the tomato paste, stock, and salt and pepper to taste.
5. Bring the mixture to a boil, then reduce the heat, cover, and simmer for 20 minutes.
6. Add the green and red bell peppers, carrot, and turnip, and cook for an additional 10 minutes.
7. In a small bowl, mix the cornstarch with 2 tablespoons of water. Add to the stew, and continue cooking for 3 minutes, stirring often. Serve warm.

Beef Moussaka

MAKES 4 SERVINGS
Preparation time: 20 minutes
Cooking time: 40 minutes

¼ teaspoon vegetable oil

1¼ pounds 95% lean ground beef

2 garlic cloves, crushed

15 fresh mint leaves, very finely chopped

¾ cup tomato paste

1 cup canned crushed tomatoes

2 eggplant, cut lengthwise and then into ½-inch slices

1 cup fat-free plain Greek-style yogurt

Salt and freshly ground black pepper

1. Preheat oven to 400°F.
2. Add ⅛ teaspoon of the oil to a small baking dish, using a paper towel to coat it and to wipe out any excess.
3. Heat a large nonstick skillet over medium heat. Add the beef and cook until browned, stirring continuously, about 5 minutes.
4. Add the garlic, mint, tomato paste, and crushed tomatoes.
5. Reduce the heat, cover, and simmer for 20 minutes, stirring occasionally.
6. Heat a medium heavy-bottomed pan over medium heat. Add the remaining ⅛ teaspoon of oil and wipe out any excess with a paper towel.
7. In batches, add the eggplant slices and cook them for 3 minutes on each side, then remove them from the pan and set aside.
8. Add the yogurt to the meat mixture and stir until combined. Season with salt and pepper.
9. On the bottom of the prepared baking dish arrange a third of the eggplant, top with half of the meat mixture, and repeat, ending with a layer of eggplant.
10. Bake for 10 minutes and serve hot.

Steak with Raspberry Vinegar and Zucchini

MAKES 4 SERVINGS

Preparation time: 30 minutes

Cooking time: 35 minutes

⅛ teaspoon vegetable oil

3 garlic cloves, chopped

1 onion, chopped

4 medium zucchini, cut into strips

1¼ pounds lean beef, such as sirloin tip or flank steak, cut into small, thin, equal-size pieces

⅓ cup raspberry vinegar

2 sprigs of fresh parsley, chopped

½ bunch of fresh tarragon, chopped

Salt and freshly ground black pepper

1. Place a nonstick, heavy-bottomed skillet over medium heat. Add the oil and wipe out any excess with a paper towel.
2. Add the garlic, onion, and zucchini and cook until browned, stirring often, about 5 minutes.
3. Add 1 cup of water, reduce the heat, cover, and simmer for 20 minutes.
4. Remove the zucchini mixture from the skillet and set aside.
5. Return the skillet to the stove and increase the heat to high. Add the meat and sear, stirring continuously, for 5 minutes. Pour in the vinegar and combine thoroughly.
6. Add the vegetables to the meat mixture, and simmer for 5 minutes.
7. Before serving, season with the parsley and tarragon, plus salt and pepper to taste.

Spicy Stuffed Zucchini

MAKES 4 SERVINGS

Preparation time: 10 minutes

Cooking time: 35 minutes

4 zucchini, cut in half lengthwise, stems removed, flesh
scooped out

Salt and freshly ground black pepper

1 pound 2 ounces 95% lean ground beef

1 cup salsa verde (a Mexican sauce made from green tomatoes
and chilies)

1 cup fat-free plain Greek-style yogurt

1. Preheat oven to 375°F.
2. Season the zucchini with salt and pepper to taste.
3. Heat a nonstick frying pan over medium heat, add the meat,
   and cook, stirring often, until browned, about 5 minutes.
4. Add the salsa and yogurt.
5. Fill the hollowed-out zucchini with the meat mixture, place
   on a baking sheet, and bake for 30 minutes.

Veal Cutlets with Lemony Grated Carrots

MAKES 4 SERVINGS

Preparation time: 15 minutes

Cooking time: 20 minutes

8 medium carrots, grated

¼ teaspoon vegetable oil

Grated zest and juice of 1 lemon

1½ pounds veal, divided into 4 portions and pounded into
⅛-inch-thick cutlets

1. Bring a pot of water to a boil, blanch the carrots for 3 minutes, drain, and cool.

2. Heat a heavy-bottomed skillet over medium heat. Add ⅛ teaspoon of the oil and wipe out any excess with a paper towel.

3. Place the carrots and lemon zest in the skillet, cover with a sheet of parchment paper, and cook for 5 minutes.

4. Remove the parchment paper and add the lemon juice. Remove the pan from the heat.

5. Heat a nonstick skillet over medium heat. Add the remaining ⅛ teaspoon of oil and wipe out any excess with a paper towel.

6. Add the veal and brown, about 1 to 3 minutes on each side.

7. Add the carrots and juices from the first skillet to the veal.

8. Heat and serve.

Oven-Baked Veal Parcels

MAKES 4 SERVINGS
Preparation time: 15 minutes
Cooking time: 30 minutes

1 onion, thinly sliced
1 carrot, thinly sliced
1 leek (white part only), thinly sliced
Salt and freshly ground black pepper
4 tablespoons of chopped fresh herbs, singly or mixed, such as
  parsley, thyme, chives
1½ pounds veal filets, split into 4 portions

1. Preheat oven to 350°F.

2. Prepare four 8 × 8-inch squares of aluminum foil.

3. In a medium saucepan, combine the onion, carrot, and leek, 2 tablespoons of water, and salt and pepper to taste.

4. Cover and cook over low heat until the vegetables are tender, about 6 minutes.

5. In the center of each square of foil, place a quarter of the vegetables, a quarter of the herbs, and a veal filet.

6. Seal up the parcels and bake on a baking sheet for 20 minutes.

Veal Niçoise

MAKES 4 SERVINGS
Preparation time: 30 minutes
Cooking time: 1 hour 50 minutes

1 pound 4 ounces firm tomatoes
2 medium carrots, sliced
2 medium onions, sliced
1 garlic clove, chopped
½ lemon, cut into four slices
1 bouquet garni (make your own by tying together 6 sprigs of
    fresh parsley, 3 sprigs of fresh thyme, and 3 dried
    bay leaves)
1 pound 9 ounces shin of veal or veal shank, cut into 4 portions
Salt and freshly ground black pepper
1 level tablespoon tomato paste

1. Fill a pot with water and bring to a boil. Add the tomatoes
   and poach for 30 seconds. Remove the tomatoes from the
   pot, peel off the skin, and remove the seeds.
2. Cut the tomatoes into large pieces.
3. In a casserole, combine the carrots and onions with 1 cup of
   water and bring to a boil.
4. Add the tomatoes, garlic, lemon, and bouquet garni. Return
   the mixture to a boil and stir.
5. Add the veal and season with salt and pepper to taste.
6. Cover and cook over low heat until the meat is tender, about
   1 hour 30 minutes.
7. Remove the bouquet garni, add the tomato paste, and season
   again with salt and pepper to taste.
8. Serve the veal with the vegetables and sauce.

Osso Bucco

MAKES 4 SERVINGS

Preparation time: 15 minutes

Cooking time: 1 hour 45 minutes

2¼ pounds shin of veal or veal shank, sliced into 4 portions

2½ tablespoons tomato paste

8 medium carrots, sliced

Grated zest and juice of 1 lemon

Grated zest of 1 orange

1 pinch of dried oregano

Salt and freshly ground black pepper

1. Turn oven on to Broil and preheat for 5 minutes.
2. Place the veal slices in a single layer on a baking sheet lined with parchment and broil until brown on both sides, about 3 minutes per side.
3. In a small bowl, combine the tomato paste and 2¼ cups of water, and mix until smooth.
4. In a heatproof casserole, combine the carrots, lemon zest, lemon juice, orange zest, tomato paste mixture, and oregano. Add salt and pepper to taste.
5. Bring the mixture to a simmer and add the veal slices.
6. Reduce the heat, cover, and simmer for 1 hour 30 minutes.

Veal Meat Loaf

MAKES 4 SERVINGS
Preparation time: 10 minutes
Cooking time: 1 hour

1 pound 10 ounces lean ground veal
4 medium carrots, grated
1 onion, chopped
1 garlic clove, chopped
7 ounces mushrooms, sliced
1¼ cups fat-free plain Greek-style yogurt
Salt and freshly ground black pepper

1. Preheat oven to 350°F.
2. In a large bowl, combine the veal, carrots, onion, garlic, mushrooms, yogurt, and salt and pepper to taste.
3. Place the mixture in a 9-inch loaf pan and bake for 1 hour.
4. Slice and serve, hot or cold.

Note: You will need a 9-inch loaf pan for this recipe.

Egg-Stuffed Veal Rolls

MAKES 2 SERVINGS

Preparation time: 20 minutes

Cooking time: 1 hour 5 minutes

2 eggs

7 ounces veal, divided into 2 portions and pounded into
⅛-inch-thick cutlets

Salt and freshly ground black pepper

1 small onion, finely chopped

3 ounces button mushrooms, finely chopped

3 sprigs of fresh thyme

1 small dried bay leaf

2¼ cups low-sodium tomato juice

1. Preheat oven to 375°F.
2. Place the eggs in a large pot and cover with cold water. Bring to a boil. Once the water is boiling, reduce the heat to a simmer and cook the eggs for 10 minutes.
3. Remove the eggs from the hot water, and help them to cool by running cold water over them. Remove the shells.
4. Season the veal with salt to taste. Then roll each hard-boiled egg up inside one wide, flat cutlet, tying each roll closed with butcher's twine.
5. Place the rolls in a small baking dish and add the onion, mushrooms, thyme, bay leaf, and tomato juice, plus salt and pepper to taste.
6. Cover the dish with a lid or foil, and bake for 45 minutes.
7. To serve, remove the string, cut each roll in half across the width, and top with the onion and mushroom sauce. Remove the bay leaf.

Roast Veal with Baby Onions

MAKES 4 TO 6 SERVINGS

Preparation time: 30 minutes

Cooking time: 50 minutes

⅛ teaspoon vegetable oil

2 medium carrots, thinly sliced

1 large onion, thinly sliced

1 garlic clove, thinly sliced

2 shallots, thinly sliced

2¼ pounds veal roast

Salt and freshly ground black pepper

20 baby onions

2 cloves

1. Preheat oven to 425°F.
2. Add the oil to a 9 × 9-inch baking dish, using a paper towel to coat it and to wipe out any excess.
3. Arrange the carrots, sliced onion, garlic, and shallots in the bottom of the dish and place the veal on top.
4. Season with salt and pepper to taste, and add 1 cup of water.
5. Cook until the veal is brown, about 20 minutes.
6. Remove the veal from the oven, and add the baby onions and cloves. Reduce the temperature to 375°F.
7. Return the veal to the oven and cook for an additional 30 minutes.

Sautéed Veal Paprika

MAKES 4 SERVINGS

Preparation time: 30 minutes

Cooking time: 30 minutes

1¾ pounds veal top round, cut into ½-inch cubes

Salt and freshly ground black pepper

⅛ teaspoon vegetable oil

1 large onion, very finely chopped

2 teaspoons paprika

2 carrots, cut into thin strips

1 large zucchini, stem removed, cut into long strips

2 tomatoes, seeds and juice removed, diced

1 cup fat-free plain Greek-style yogurt

1. Preheat oven to 375°F.
2. Season the veal with salt and pepper to taste. Heat a large, heavy-bottomed ovenproof skillet over medium heat. Add the oil and wipe out any excess with a paper towel.
3. Place the veal in the skillet and brown, stirring often, about 5 minutes.
4. Mix in the onion and paprika.
5. Place the veal in the oven and cook for 20 minutes.
6. While the veal is cooking, fill the bottom part of a large steamer halfway with water and bring to a simmer.
7. Place the carrots, zucchini, and tomatoes in the top part of the steamer, cover, and cook for 5 minutes.
8. Remove the veal from the oven, stir in the yogurt, and add more salt and pepper to taste.
9. To serve, transfer the veal to a serving dish and arrange the vegetables around it.

Note: You will need a steamer for this recipe.

Veal Chops

MAKES 2 SERVINGS

Preparation time: 15 minutes

Cooking time: 45 minutes

⅛ teaspoon vegetable oil

1¼ cups no-salt-added canned diced tomatoes

1 carrot, grated

1 stalk of celery, chopped

1 teaspoon finely chopped fresh basil

Salt and freshly ground black pepper

2 veal chops, about 5 ounces each

1. Preheat oven to 350°F.
2. Add the oil to a small ovenproof dish, using a paper towel to coat it and to wipe out any excess.
3. In a medium bowl, combine the tomatoes, carrot, celery, and basil. Add salt and pepper to taste.
4. Place half the vegetable mixture on the bottom of the prepared ovenproof dish, layer the meat on top, and finish with the remaining vegetables.
5. Bake for 45 minutes.

Veal in Tomato Herb Sauce

MAKES 4 SERVINGS

Preparation time: 10 minutes

Cooking time: 45 minutes

⅛ teaspoon vegetable oil

2 pounds 4 ounces veal roast

Salt and freshly ground black pepper

1 low-sodium veal or beef bouillon cube

1 garlic clove, finely chopped

1 large shallot, finely chopped

1 tablespoon herbes de Provence (a mix of dried marjoram,
    thyme, savory, basil, rosemary, sage, and fennel seeds)

1 tomato, stem removed, cut into pieces

1. Preheat oven to 375°F.
2. Add the oil to a heatproof casserole, using a paper towel to coat it and to wipe out any excess.
3. Season the veal with salt and pepper to taste, and brown in the casserole on all sides, about 5 minutes.
4. Place the casserole in the oven and cook the veal until the internal temperature reaches 150°F, about 30 minutes.
5. Remove the veal from the casserole and set it aside to rest.
6. Add 1 cup of boiling water and the bouillon cube to the casserole and stir until the cube is dissolved.
7. Add the garlic, shallot, and herbs to the broth, along with salt and pepper to taste.
8. Cook over low heat until the sauce is slightly reduced, about 10 minutes.
9. Add the tomato. Serve the veal sliced with the sauce.

Calf's Liver with Tomato

MAKES 1 SERVING

Preparation time: 20 minutes

Cooking time: 20 minutes

3½ ounces calf's liver

⅛ teaspoon vegetable oil

1 medium onion, thinly sliced

1 large tomato, chopped or 1 cup of canned no-salt-added diced
tomatoes

½ teaspoon dried oregano

1 teaspoon cornstarch

Salt and freshly ground black pepper

2 tablespoons chopped fresh flat-leaf parsley

1. Slice the calf's liver diagonally to produce three or four very
   thin, small slices.
2. Heat a nonstick frying pan over medium heat, add the oil to
   coat, and remove excess with a paper towel.
3. Add onion and cook until lightly browned, stirring often,
   about 3 minutes. Remove the onion from the pan and set it
   aside.
4. Using the same frying pan, cook the tomato, with the oregano, stirring often for about 3 minutes.
5. Remove the tomato from the pan and set it aside. Coat the
   calf's liver slices with cornstarch and season with salt and
   pepper to taste.
6. Cook the liver in the same pan until browned on both sides,
   about 2 minutes per side.
7. To serve, place the slices of liver on a plate with the tomato
   and onion, and garnish with parsley. Serve hot.

Ham Tart

MAKES 4 SERVINGS
Preparation time: 15 minutes
Cooking time: 30 minutes

⅛ teaspoon vegetable oil

3 tablespoons cornstarch

2 eggs, separated

1 cup fat-free plain Greek-style yogurt

3 ounces fat-free cream cheese (optional)

4 shallots, very finely chopped

Salt and freshly ground black pepper

7 ounces extra-lean ham, chopped

2 tomatoes, thinly sliced

1. Preheat oven to 425°F.
2. Add the oil to a 9-inch pie dish, using a paper towel to coat it and to wipe out any excess.
3. In a medium bowl, combine the cornstarch, egg yolks, yogurt, and cream cheese (if using).
4. In a mixing bowl, beat the egg whites until stiff.
5. Fold the egg whites into the yogurt mixture.
6. Fill the prepared pie dish with the egg mixture.
7. Top with the shallots, season with salt and pepper to taste, then arrange the ham and tomato slices on top.
8. Bake for 25 to 30 minutes. Serve hot or cold.

Tarragon Rabbit

MAKES 4 SERVINGS
Preparation time: 20 minutes
Cooking time: 55 minutes

⅛ teaspoon vegetable oil

1 pound button mushrooms, sliced

1 rabbit or a 3½-pound chicken (skin removed), cut into pieces

1 tablespoon chopped shallots

2 teaspoons chopped garlic

10 sprigs of fresh tarragon, leaves removed and saved, stems discarded

1 sprig of fresh thyme

1 dried bay leaf

3 tablespoons raspberry vinegar

Salt and freshly ground black pepper

2 tablespoons fat-free plain Greek-style yogurt

1. Heat oven to 375°F.
2. Heat a large heatproof casserole over medium heat. Add the oil and wipe out any excess with a paper towel.
3. Add the mushrooms and the rabbit and cook, stirring often, until browned, about 8 minutes.
4. Add the shallots, garlic, half the tarragon leaves, and the thyme, bay leaf, and vinegar, plus salt and pepper to taste.
5. Cover and bake until the rabbit is cooked through, about 30 minutes.
6. Remove the rabbit from the casserole and reduce the sauce over medium heat, about 5 minutes.
7. Add the yogurt and the remaining tarragon to the sauce, and mix until thoroughly combined. Remove the bay leaf.
8. Serve the rabbit with the sauce.

Rabbit Terrine

MAKES 4 SERVINGS

Preparation time: 25 minutes, plus 2 hours for refrigeration
Cooking time: 1 hour 40 minutes

1 pound boneless rabbit meat (or an equal amount of chicken), chopped

4 slices of extra-lean ham (or cooked chicken), chopped

1 white onion, chopped

3 shallots, chopped

2 eggs, beaten

2 sprigs of fresh parsley, chopped

Salt and freshly ground black pepper

4 large lettuce leaves

1. Preheat oven to 350°F.
2. Fill the bottom part of a large steamer halfway with water and bring to a simmer.
3. Place the rabbit in the top part of the steamer, cover, and cook for 10 minutes.
4. Place the rabbit, ham, onion, and shallots in a food processor and pulse on and off until you have very small, even pieces.
5. Add the beaten eggs, parsley, and salt and pepper to taste, and process until thoroughly combined.
6. Transfer the mixture to a 9-inch loaf pan. Place the loaf pan into a bigger baking dish and fill this dish halfway with cold water.
7. Place the baking dish into the oven and bake for 1½ hours.
8. Remove the loaf pan from the oven, cool, cover, and refrigerate until cold, about 2 hours.
9. Serve slices of terrine atop a bed of lettuce, seasoned with salt and pepper to taste.

Note: You will need a large steamer and a 9-inch loaf pan for this recipe.

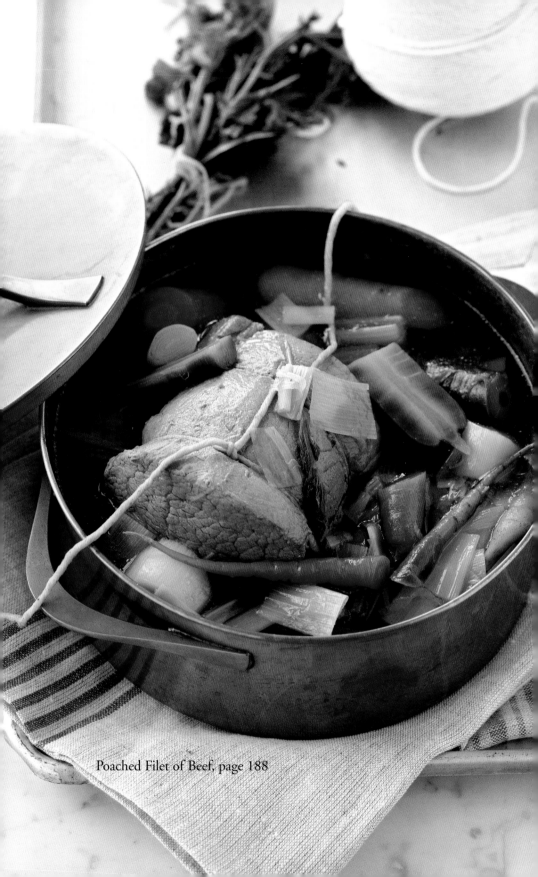

Poached Filet of Beef, page 188

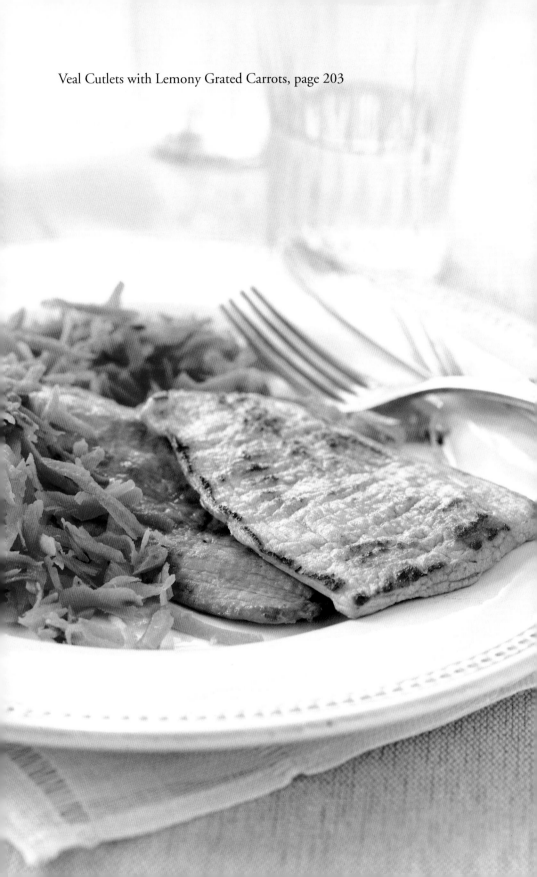

Veal Cutlets with Lemony Grated Carrots, page 203

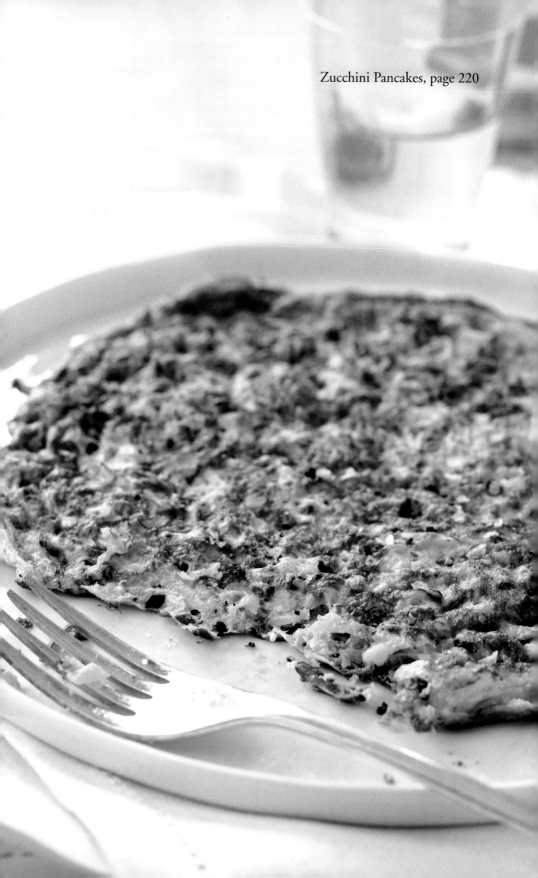
Zucchini Pancakes, page 220

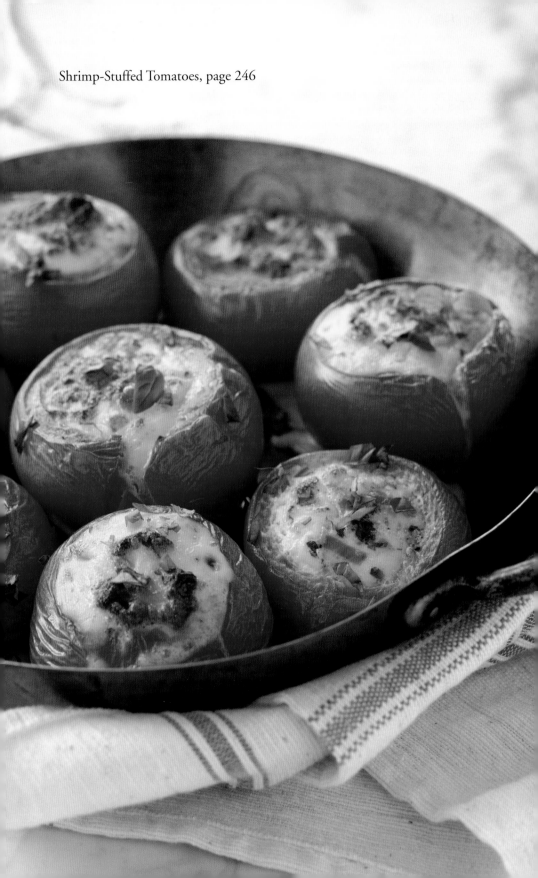

Shrimp-Stuffed Tomatoes, page 246

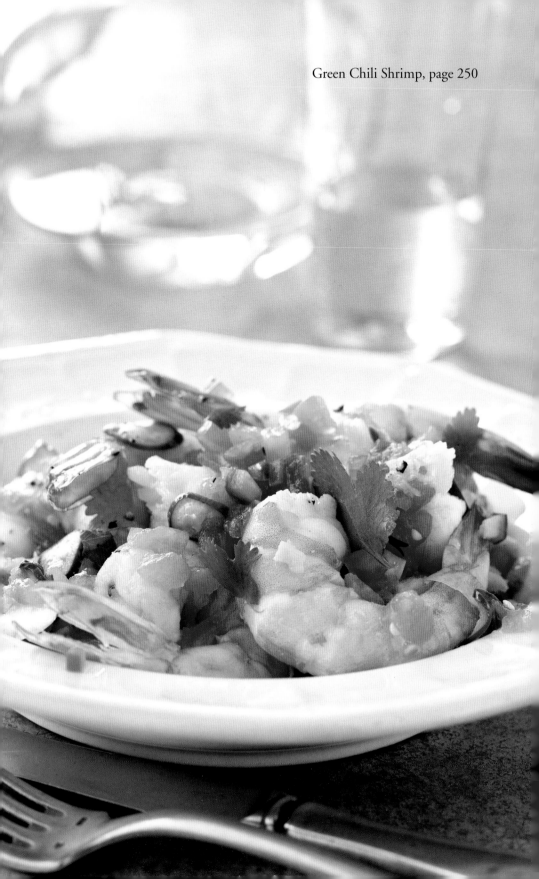

Green Chili Shrimp, page 250

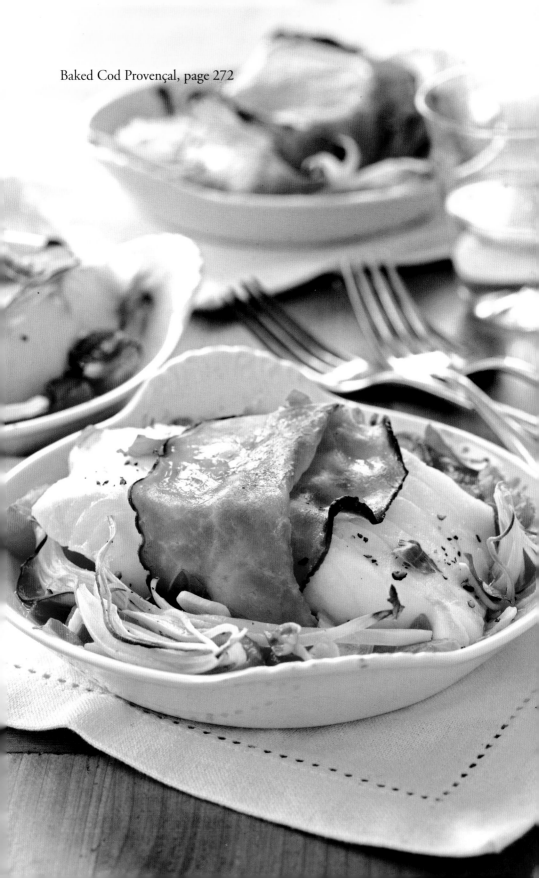

Baked Cod Provençal, page 272

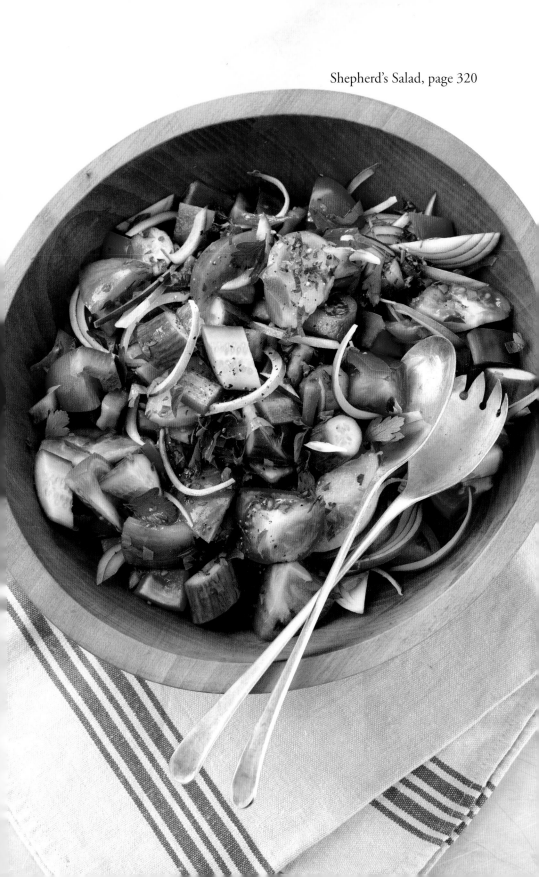
Shepherd's Salad, page 320

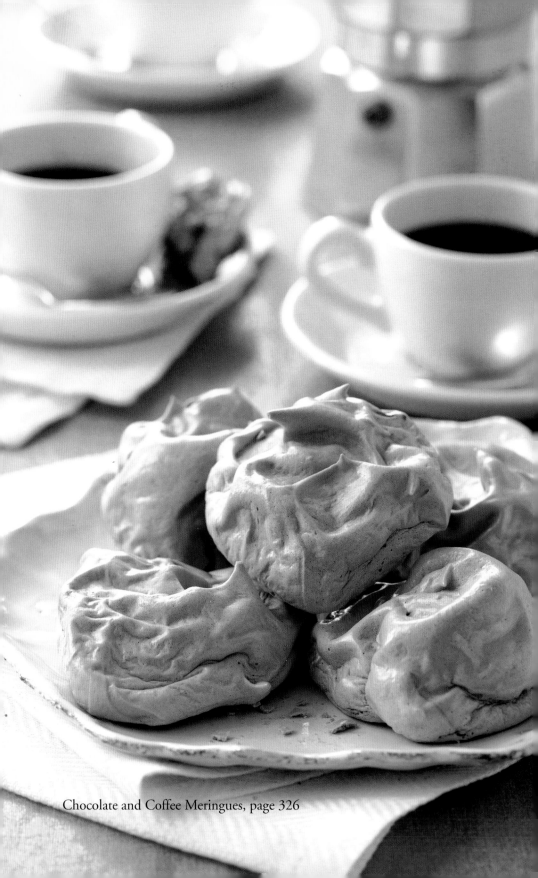

Chocolate and Coffee Meringues, page 326

Spinach- Ham- and Turkey-Stuffed Mushrooms

MAKES 2 SERVINGS

Preparation time: 25 minutes

Cooking time: 25 minutes

1 low-sodium veal or low-sodium beef bouillon cube

4 ounces spinach

14 ounces large button mushrooms (big enough to stuff)

Juice of 1 lemon

1 garlic clove, chopped

1 slice of extra-lean ham, chopped

2 slices of cooked turkey, chopped

2 tablespoons chopped fresh parsley

1 tablespoon oat bran, such as Dukan Diet Organic Oat Bran

3 to 4 tablespoons fat-free milk

Salt and freshly ground black pepper

1. Preheat oven to 350°F.
2. Fill a medium pot with water and bring to a boil. Add the bouillon cube.
3. Blanch the spinach for 2 minutes, remove, drain, and set aside.
4. Separate the mushroom tops from the stalks. Sprinkle the lemon juice over the tops and set aside. Finely chop the stalks.
5. Squeeze the excess water out of the spinach and chop thoroughly.
6. In a medium bowl, combine the spinach, mushroom stalks, garlic, ham, turkey, parsley, oat bran, and milk, plus salt and pepper to taste.
7. Stuff the mushroom tops with the spinach mixture.
8. Place the stuffed mushrooms on a baking sheet lined with parchment and bake for 20 minutes.

Discover Dukan Diet Organic Oat Bran

Eggs and Vegetables

Tofu Omelet

MAKES 4 SERVINGS
Preparation time: 15 minutes
Cooking time: 10 minutes

2 eggs
2 tablespoons low-sodium soy sauce
1 garlic clove, finely chopped
½ onion, chopped
Freshly ground black pepper
14 ounces firm tofu, cut into small cubes
½ green bell pepper, seeds removed, chopped
⅛ teaspoon vegetable oil
1 tablespoon chopped fresh parsley

1. In a medium bowl, beat the eggs, soy sauce, garlic, and onion until thoroughly combined. Add black pepper to taste.
2. Add the tofu and green pepper and mix thoroughly.
3. Heat an 8-inch or heavy-bottomed cast-iron skillet over medium heat. Add the oil and wipe out any excess with a paper towel.
4. Pour the omelet mixture into the skillet, reduce the heat, cover, and cook until firm, about 10 minutes.
5. Serve topped with the chopped parsley.

Zucchini and Ham Loaf

MAKES 4 SERVINGS

Preparation time: 25 minutes

Cooking time: 20 minutes

1 pound zucchini, thinly sliced

Salt and freshly ground black pepper

4 eggs

4 ounces extra-lean ham

1 tablespoon fat-free ricotta

1 tablespoon fat-free plain Greek-style yogurt

1 tablespoon fat-free cream cheese (optional)

A pinch of ground nutmeg

1 tablespoon cornstarch

¼ cup fat-free milk

1. Line a microwave-proof loaf pan with parchment paper.
2. Place the zucchini in a microwave-proof dish (not the pan you have lined with paper). Add 3 tablespoons of water and microwave for 5 minutes on the maximum setting.
3. Drain the zucchini, season with salt and pepper to taste, and place in a blender with the eggs, ham, ricotta, yogurt, cream cheese (if using), and nutmeg, plus salt and pepper to taste. Process until smooth, about 30 seconds. Transfer processed zucchini mixture into a large bowl.
4. In a small bowl, combine the cornstarch with 2 tablespoons of cold water and the milk.
5. Stir the cornstarch mixture into the zucchini mixture.
6. Pour the zucchini mixture into the prepared loaf pan and cover.
7. Cook for 15 minutes in the microwave, then leave to rest for 5 minutes before taking it out of the microwave. Serve warm or cool.

Zucchini Pancakes

MAKES 3 SERVINGS
Preparation time: 15 minutes
Cooking time: 15 minutes

6 eggs, separated
4 medium zucchini, very finely chopped
1 garlic clove, chopped
3 sprigs of fresh parsley, chopped
Salt and freshly ground black pepper
⅛ teaspoon vegetable oil per pancake

1. In a mixing bowl, beat the egg whites until stiff.
2. In a medium bowl, mix the zucchini with the egg yolks, garlic, and parsley, plus salt and pepper to taste. Gently fold in the egg whites.
3. Heat a heavy-bottomed or a cast iron skillet over medium heat. Add ⅛ teaspoon of the oil and wipe out any excess with a paper towel.
4. Drop a third of the batter into the skillet at a time, and cook about 3 minutes on each side. Repeat the oiling procedure for each batch.

Tuna and Zucchini Frittata

MAKES 4 SERVINGS
Preparation time: 20 minutes, plus 1 hour for cooling
Cooking time: 20 minutes

3 thin zucchini, diced
Salt and freshly ground black pepper
1 white onion, thinly sliced
6 eggs, beaten
1 (5-ounce) can of tuna packed in water
⅛ teaspoon vegetable oil
2 tablespoons balsamic vinegar

1. Fill the bottom part of a large steamer halfway with water and bring to a simmer.
2. Place the zucchini in the top part of the steamer, cover, and cook for 5 minutes.
3. Remove the zucchini from the steamer and season with salt and pepper to taste.
4. In a medium bowl, combine the zucchini, onion, eggs, and tuna, plus more salt and pepper to taste, if desired.
5. Heat a medium nonstick skillet over medium heat. Add the oil and wipe out any excess with a paper towel.
6. Pour the omelet mixture into the skillet, stir, reduce the heat, and cover.
7. Cook the omelet over low heat until the eggs are set, about 10 minutes.
8. Let cool for 1 hour, cut into small slices, and season with vinegar when ready to serve.

Note: You will need a large steamer for this recipe.

Endive Frittata

MAKES 4 SERVINGS
Preparation time: 15 minutes
Cooking time: 25 minutes

⅛ teaspoon vegetable oil
2¼ pounds endive
Salt and freshly ground black pepper
4 eggs, beaten
⅔ cup fat-free milk
A pinch of grated nutmeg

1. Preheat oven to 375°F.
2. Add the oil to a small baking dish, using a paper towel to coat it and to wipe out any excess.
3. Separate the endive leaves and discard the stem.

4. Fill a pot with hot water, add a pinch of salt, and bring to a boil. Blanch the endive in the boiling water for 2 minutes, then drain.

5. In a medium bowl, combine the eggs, milk, and nutmeg, plus salt and pepper to taste.

6. Place the endive leaves in the prepared baking dish and pour the egg mixture over them.

7. Bake until the eggs have set, about 20 minutes.

Baked Endive and Eggs

MAKES 2 SERVINGS

Preparation time: 20 minutes

Cooking time: 45 minutes

¼ teaspoon vegetable oil

3 eggs

2 onions, finely chopped

14 ounces endive

Salt and freshly ground black pepper

1¾ cups low-sodium tomato juice

1. Preheat oven to 425°F.

2. Add ⅛ teaspoon of the oil to a 9 × 9-inch baking dish, using a paper towel to coat it and to wipe out any excess.

3. Place the eggs in a large pot, cover with cold water, and bring to a boil. Once the water is boiling, reduce to a simmer and cook the eggs for 10 minutes.

4. Remove the eggs from the pot and cool them by running cold water over them. Remove the shells and chop the eggs.

5. Heat a heavy-bottomed or a cast-iron skillet over medium heat. Add the remaining ⅛ teaspoon of oil and wipe out any excess with a paper towel.

6. Add the onions and cook until brown, about 5 minutes.

7. Fill the bottom part of a large steamer halfway with water and bring to a simmer.

8. Separate the endive leaves and discard the stem.

9. Place the endive in the top part of the steamer, cover, and cook for 5 minutes, then remove.

10. Fill the prepared baking dish with the endive leaves and onions, top with the eggs, and add salt and pepper to taste. Pour the tomato juice over the top.

11. Bake for 15 minutes.

Note: You will need a steamer for this recipe.

Cucumber in Yogurt Sauce

MAKES 2 SERVINGS
Preparation time: 10 minutes
Cooking time: No cooking required

1 cup fat-free plain Greek-style yogurt
½ cucumber, peeled and cut into ½-inch cubes
½ garlic clove, crushed
Juice of ½ lemon
Salt and freshly ground black pepper
¼ yellow or green bell pepper, seeds removed and cut into very thin strips
1 red bell pepper, seeds removed, cut into very thin strips

1. In a medium bowl, mix the yogurt, cucumber, garlic, and lemon juice until thoroughly combined. Season with salt and pepper to taste.

2. Serve with the strips of bell pepper.

Cucumber and Basil Soufflé

MAKES 2 SERVINGS
Preparation time: 20 minutes
Cooking time: 35 minutes

Salt and freshly ground black pepper
4 tomatoes, with stems removed
¼ teaspoon vegetable oil
2 onions, thinly sliced
½ bunch of fresh basil
½ cucumber, peeled and seeded
¼ cup fat-free plain Greek-style yogurt
6 egg whites

1. Preheat oven to 400°F.
2. Fill a medium pot with water, add a pinch of salt, and bring to a boil. Poach the tomatoes for 30 seconds. Remove the tomatoes from the pot, peel off the skin, remove the seeds, and cut into small cubes.
3. Heat a nonstick skillet over medium heat. Add ⅛ teaspoon of the oil and wipe out any excess with a paper towel. Place the onions into the the skillet and cook, stirring often until soft, about 5 minutes.
4. Reduce the heat, add the tomatoes to the skillet, season with salt and pepper to taste, and cook for 15 minutes. Remove the mixture from the heat and set aside.
5. Pull the basil leaves off the stems and discard the stems.
6. In a blender, process the cucumber, yogurt, and 8 basil leaves until puréed, about 30 seconds. Season with salt and pepper to taste and transfer to a large bowl.
7. In a mixing bowl, beat the egg whites until stiff and fold them into the cucumber mixture.
8. Coat two 2-cup ramekins with the remaining ⅛ teaspoon of oil, and remove any excess with a paper towel.
9. Place half the tomato mixture into each ramekin, then pour the soufflé mixture into each ramekin until it is two-thirds full.

10. Bake for 15 minutes. Once the soufflés are cooked, garnish each with a basil leaf.

Note: You will need two 2-cup ramekins for this recipe.

Baked Eggs with Tomato Basil Sauce

MAKES 2 SERVINGS
Preparation time: 10 minutes
Cooking time: 40 minutes

4 eggs
¾ cup fat-free milk
A pinch of ground nutmeg
Salt and freshly ground black pepper
⅛ teaspoon vegetable oil
6 tomatoes, stems and seeds removed, diced
3 basil leaves

1. Preheat oven to 350°F.
2. In a medium bowl, beat the eggs with the milk, nutmeg, and salt and pepper to taste.
3. Coat two 1-cup ramekins with the oil and wipe out any excess with a paper towel. Fill with the egg mixture.
4. Place the ramekins in a bigger baking dish and fill the baking dish halfway with cold water. Bake for 40 minutes.
5. While the egg mixture is baking, place the tomatoes, basil, and salt and pepper to taste in a medium pot and cook over medium heat, stirring occasionally until it becomes a thick sauce, about 20 minutes.
6. Turn the baked eggs out of the ramekins and pour the sauce over them. Serve hot.

Note: You will need two 1-cup ramekins for this recipe.

Stuffed Baked Tomatoes

MAKES 4 SERVINGS
Preparation time: 15 minutes
Cooking time: 25 minutes

8 tomatoes
Salt and freshly ground black pepper
4 eggs
7 ounces extra-lean ham, finely chopped
2 tablespoons very finely chopped fresh basil

1. Preheat oven to 425°F.
2. Cut the tops off the tomatoes, spoon out the insides, sprinkle a little salt inside, and turn them over on a plate to let their juices drain.
3. In a medium bowl, beat the eggs, season with salt and pepper to taste, and add the ham and basil.
4. Turn the tomatoes over and place them in a baking dish. Spoon the egg mixture into the tomatoes and bake for 25 minutes.

Eggplant Frittata

MAKES 2 SERVINGS
Preparation time: 20 minutes, plus 30 minutes for the eggplant juices to drain
Cooking time: 35 minutes

14 ounces eggplant, peeled and cut into ½-inch slices
Salt and freshly ground black pepper
3 eggs
1 cup fat-free milk
A pinch of ground nutmeg
3 sprigs of fresh thyme, chopped
3 sprigs of fresh rosemary, chopped
⅛ teaspoon vegetable oil

1. Preheat oven to 300°F.
2. Place the eggplant slices in a colander, sprinkle them with a little salt and set them aside until their juices drain out, about 30 minutes.
3. Wipe the slices dry with a clean kitchen towel.
4. Bring a medium pot of water to a boil and blanch the eggplant for 5 minutes, then drain.
5. In a medium bowl, mix the eggs, milk, nutmeg, thyme, rosemary, and salt and pepper to taste until thoroughly combined.
6. Coat a 9 × 9-inch baking dish with the oil and wipe out any excess with a paper towel.
7. Arrange the eggplant slices in the prepared baking dish and pour the egg mixture over the eggplant.
8. Bake for 30 minutes.

Omelets with Anchovy Sauce

MAKES 4 SERVINGS
Preparation time: 15 minutes
Cooking time: 25 minutes

3 tomatoes, stems removed and quartered
8 canned anchovies, rinsed, dried, and chopped
1 tablespoon capers, drained and rinsed
8 eggs
2 tablespoons fat-free milk
10 fresh chives, finely chopped
5 sprigs of fresh cilantro, finely chopped
5 sprigs of fresh parsley, finely chopped
Salt and freshly ground black pepper
⅜ teaspoon vegetable oil, divided
6 sun-dried tomatoes, rehydrated and chopped

1. Heat a nonstick skillet over medium heat. Add ⅛ teaspoon of the oil and wipe out any excess with a paper towel. Add the tomatoes, anchovies, and capers.

2. Cook, stirring often, for 5 minutes. Transfer the sauce to a small bowl and set aside.

3. In a medium bowl, beat together the eggs, milk, chives, cilantro, and parsley, plus salt and pepper to taste.

4. Reheat the skillet over medium heat, coat with ⅛ teaspoon of the oil, and wipe out any excess with a paper towel.

5. Pour in half the egg mixture and cook the eggs until set, about 10 minutes.

6. Transfer the omelet to a plate. Repeat with the remaining oil and the rest of the egg mixture.

7. Let the omelets cool, then cut them into strips ¾ inch wide.

8. Place the omelet strips in a shallow bowl, add the sauce and the sun-dried tomatoes, and gently toss until well combined. Serve warm.

Mushroom Soufflé

MAKES 1 SERVING
Preparation time: 15 minutes
Cooking time: 20 minutes

⅛ teaspoon vegetable oil
⅔ cup button mushrooms
1 egg, separated
1 egg white
3 tablespoons fat-free plain Greek-style yogurt
Salt and freshly ground black pepper

1. Preheat oven to 350°F.

2. Add oil to 1½-cup ramekin and wipe out any excess with a paper towel.

3. Bring a medium pot of water to a boil and blanch the mushrooms for 2 minutes, then drain.

4. In a mixing bowl, beat the 2 egg whites until stiff.

5. In a blender, process the mushrooms, egg yolk, and yogurt until smooth, about 45 seconds.

6. Transfer the mushroom mixture to a medium bowl and fold in the egg whites. Season with salt and pepper to taste.

7. Pour the mixture into the prepared ramekin and bake until lightly browned on top, about 15 minutes.

Note: You will need one 1½-cup ramekin for this recipe.

Mushroom Tart

MAKES 2 SERVINGS
Preparation time: 15 minutes
Cooking time: 40 minutes

⅛ teaspoon vegetable oil

3 eggs

2 cups fat-free milk

2 teaspoons active dry yeast

Salt and freshly ground black pepper

1 small green bell pepper, seeds removed, chopped into very small pieces

1 zucchini, chopped into very small pieces

4 large button mushrooms, chopped into very small pieces

1 small onion, chopped into very small pieces

1. Preheat oven to 450°F.

2. Add the oil to a 9 × 9-inch baking dish, using a paper towel to coat it and to wipe out any excess.

3. In a medium bowl, whisk together the eggs, milk, and yeast, plus salt and pepper to taste. Let sit for 5 minutes.

4. Add the bell pepper, zucchini, mushrooms, and onion.

5. Pour the egg mixture into the prepared baking dish.

6. Bake until set, about 40 minutes.

Vegetable Tart

MAKES 2 SERVINGS
Preparation time: 10 minutes
Cooking time: 30 minutes

⅛ teaspoon vegetable oil

4 eggs

1 pinch of ground nutmeg

1 tablespoon chopped fresh herbs, singly or mixed, such as
    basil, parsley, and rosemary

2¼ cups fat-free milk

1 cup chopped mixed vegetables, such as tomatoes, zucchini,
    broccoli, eggplant, and carrots, with all stems removed

Salt and freshly ground black pepper

1. Preheat oven to 350°F.
2. Add the oil to a 9 × 9-inch baking dish, using a paper towel to coat it and to wipe out any excess.
3. In a medium bowl, combine the eggs, nutmeg, herbs, and milk.
4. Add the vegetables.
5. Fill the prepared baking dish with the egg mixture.
6. Place the dish into a larger baking dish and fill the larger dish halfway with cold water.
7. Bake for 30 minutes.

Provençal Vegetable Tart

MAKES 4 SERVINGS
Preparation time: 35 minutes
Cooking time: 45 minutes

¼ teaspoon vegetable oil

4 tomatoes, stems removed

2¼ cups finely chopped zucchini

2 red bell peppers, seeds removed, finely chopped

1 onion, thinly sliced

Salt and freshly ground black pepper

4 eggs

¼ cup fat-free milk

1 tablespoon fat-free cream cheese (optional)

1. Preheat oven to 400°F.
2. Add ⅛ teaspoon of the oil to a 9-inch nonstick loaf pan, using a paper towel to coat it and to wipe out any excess.
3. Fill a pot with water and bring to a boil. Add the tomatoes and poach for 30 seconds. Remove the tomatoes from the pot, peel off the skin, remove the seeds, and dice.
4. Heat a heavy-bottomed or a cast-iron skillet over medium heat. Add the remaining ⅛ teaspoon of oil and wipe out any excess with a paper towel.
5. Add the zucchini, bell peppers, and onion and cook, stirring often, for 10 minutes. Season with salt and pepper to taste.
6. In a medium bowl, beat together the eggs, milk, and cream cheese (if using). Season with salt and pepper to taste.
7. Add the vegetable mixture to the egg mixture and pour into the prepared loaf pan. Place the loaf pan inside a larger pan and fill the larger one halfway with water.
8. Bake for 30 minutes.

Note: You will need a 9-inch loaf pan for this recipe.

—— *Shirataki Noodles and Vegetables* ——

Shirataki noodles were developed in Asia. Made of yam starch, they are very high in fiber and very low in carbohydrates and calories, making them an ideal food for the Dukan dieter. They can be added to soups or stir-fries, integrated into any protein dish, or simply prepared like pasta and served with your favorite sauce.

The noodles need to be drained from their packaging, rinsed, and cooked before you use them in a recipe. The noodles can be bought from our website: www.shopdukandiet.com.

To prepare shirataki noodles on the stovetop:

1. Remove the noodles from their packaging, drain in a colander, and rinse thoroughly under cold running water.
2. Fill a medium saucepan with water and bring to a boil.
3. Add the noodles, return the water to a boil, and cook for 2 minutes.
4. Drain the noodles, rinse again, and pat dry with a paper towel. Use as desired.

To prepare shirataki noodles in the microwave:

1. Remove the noodles from their packaging, drain in a colander, and rinse thoroughly under cold running water.
2. Place the noodles in a microwave-safe dish and cook for 1 minute.
3. Drain the noodles, rinse again, and pat dry with a paper towel. Use as desired.

Three-Pepper Shirataki Noodles

MAKES 4 SERVINGS

Preparation time: 15 minutes, plus 30 minutes for chilling

Cooking time: 2 minutes

4 tomatoes, diced

1 red bell pepper, stem and seeds removed, diced

1 green bell pepper, stem and seeds removed, diced

1 yellow bell pepper, stem and seeds removed, diced

3 tablespoons Vinaigrette Maya (page 330)

2 tablespoons red wine vinegar

1 garlic clove, chopped

2 tablespoons finely chopped fresh parsley

½ teaspoon cayenne pepper

Salt and freshly ground black pepper to taste

2 (7-ounce) packages of shirataki noodles, such as Dukan Diet
    Shirataki Noodles, prepared according to the directions on
    page 232.

1. In a large bowl, combine the tomatoes and the red, green, and yellow bell peppers.
2. In a small bowl, combine the vinaigrette, vinegar, garlic, parsley, and cayenne pepper. Add salt and pepper to taste.
3. Add the cooked noodles to the vegetable mixture, dress with the vinaigrette, and combine thoroughly.
4. Cover and refrigerate until chilled, about 30 minutes.

Thai Chicken with Broccoli and Shirataki Noodles

4 SERVINGS

Preparation time: 15 minutes

Cooking time: 30 minutes

¼ teaspoon vegetable oil

4 boneless, skinless chicken breasts, chopped into ½-inch cubes

1 egg plus 2 egg whites, lightly beaten

2 scallions, thinly sliced

1 head of broccoli, chopped into small florets

3 garlic cloves, chopped

1 teaspoon powdered stevia extract such as Dukan Diet
Organic Stevia

1 tablespoon red wine vinegar

¼ cup fresh lime juice

Salt

1 tablespoon cornstarch

2 (7-ounce) packages of shirataki noodles, such as Dukan Diet
Shirataki Noodles, prepared according to the directions on
page 232.

1 tablespoon finely chopped fresh cilantro

Low-sodium soy sauce

Thai hot sauce, such as Sriracha (optional)

1. Heat a large nonstick skillet over medium heat. Add ⅛ teaspoon of the oil and wipe out any excess with a paper towel. Add the chicken, and cook thoroughly, stirring often, about 5 minutes.

2. Add the eggs and cook, stirring often, for an additional 3 minutes. Transfer to a dish and set aside.

3. Return the skillet to a burner and adjust the heat to low. Add the remaining oil and wipe out any excess with a paper towel.

4. Add the scallions and cook, stirring often, until soft, about 5 minutes.

5. Add the broccoli and 2 tablespoons of water.

6. Cover the skillet and cook for 5 minutes.

7. Add the garlic, stevia, vinegar, lime juice, chicken, and salt to taste. Stir until combined.

8. In a small bowl, thoroughly combine the cornstarch and 1 tablespoon of water.

9. Pour the cornstarch mixture over the broccoli and chicken, and stir it in very quickly and vigorously so that none of it sticks to the bottom of the skillet. Remove the pan from the heat.

10. To serve, divide the cooked noodles among 4 bowls and top with equal portions of the chicken mixture.

11. Garnish with chopped cilantro, and add soy sauce and hot sauce to taste.

Shirataki Noodles with Balsamic Vinegar

MAKES 4 SERVINGS

Preparation time: 5 minutes, plus 1 to 2 hours for marinating

Cooking time: 2 minutes

¼ cup balsamic vinegar

2 tablespoons chopped fresh basil

2 garlic cloves, finely chopped

Salt and freshly ground black pepper

2 tomatoes, finely diced

1 red onion, finely chopped

2 (7-ounce) packages of shirataki noodles, such as Dukan Diet Shirataki Noodles, prepared according to the directions on page 232.

1. In a large bowl, thoroughly combine the vinegar, basil, and garlic. Add salt and pepper to taste.

2. Add the tomatoes and onion, stir well, cover, and leave at room temperature to marinate for 1 to 2 hours.

3. Add the prepared noodles to the tomato mixture, and season with salt and pepper to taste before serving.

Garlic Shirataki Noodles

MAKES 4 SERVINGS

Preparation time: 10 minutes

Cooking time: 2 minutes

2 tablespoons white wine vinegar

3 tablespoons Vinaigrette Maya (page 330)

2 garlic cloves, chopped

Salt and freshly ground black pepper

4 tomatoes, very finely chopped

1 red bell pepper, stem and seeds removed, finely chopped

1 green bell pepper, stem and seeds removed, finely chopped

1 yellow bell pepper, stem and seeds removed, finely chopped

1 tablespoon capers, drained and rinsed

1 teaspoon caper brine

2 (7-ounce) packages of shirataki noodles, such as Dukan Diet
Shirataki Noodles, prepared according to the directions on
page 232.

1. In a large bowl, thoroughly combine the vinegar, vinaigrette, and garlic, plus salt and black pepper to taste.
2. Add the tomatoes, bell peppers, capers, and caper brine.
3. Place the prepared shirataki noodles in a large bowl, top with the tomato mixture, and add salt and pepper to taste.

Shirataki Noodles with Ground Beef, Cherry Tomatoes, and Asparagus

MAKES 4 SERVINGS

Preparation time: 10 minutes

Cooking time: 20 minutes

⅛ teaspoon vegetable oil

1 onion, chopped

1 pound 95% lean ground beef

Salt and freshly ground black pepper

3 ounces cherry tomatoes (about 15), cut in half

12 spears of asparagus, cut into ½-inch pieces

2 (7-ounce) packages of shirataki noodles, such as Dukan Diet Shirataki Noodles, prepared according to the directions on page 232.

1. Heat a large nonstick skillet over medium heat. Add the oil, and wipe out any excess with a paper towel.
2. Add the onion to the pan and cook, stirring often, for 5 to 6 minutes.
3. Add the ground beef and season with salt and pepper to taste.
4. Cook, stirring constantly, until browned, about 5 minutes.
5. Add the tomatoes and asparagus. Cook, stirring constantly, until the asparagus is tender, about 5 minutes.
6. Add the prepared noodles and cook, stirring constantly, for an additional 3 minutes.

Shirataki Noodles Bolognese

MAKES 2 TO 3 SERVINGS

Preparation time: 10 minutes

Cooking time: 1 hour 20 minutes

1 garlic clove, finely chopped

1 onion, finely diced

1 carrot, finely diced

1 stalk of celery, peeled and sliced

½ teaspoon finely chopped fresh thyme

½ teaspoon finely chopped fresh oregano

1 dried bay leaf

Salt and freshly ground black pepper

1 pound 95% lean ground beef

2 tomatoes, roughly chopped or 1 cup low-sodium beef stock

2 (7-ounce) packages of shirataki noodles, such as Dukan Diet
    Shirataki Noodles, prepared according to the directions on
    page 232.

1. Place a large nonstick skillet over low heat, and add 3 table-spoons of water and the garlic and onion. Cook until soft, about 2 minutes.

2. Add the carrot, celery, thyme, oregano, and bay leaf, plus salt and pepper to taste, and cook for an additional 10 minutes.

3. Add the beef and cook, stirring constantly, until browned, about 5 minutes.

4. Add the tomatoes or beef stock.

5. Bring to a boil, reduce the heat to a simmer, season with salt and pepper to taste, and cook for 1 hour.

6. Add the prepared noodles to the sauce and cook until heated thoroughly, about 5 minutes. Remove the bay leaf before serving.

Shirataki Noodles with Green Vegetables and Artichoke Hearts

MAKES 4 SERVINGS

Preparation time: 10 minutes, plus 2 hours for marinating

Cooking time: 2 minutes

5 artichoke hearts, chopped

1 cup alfalfa sprouts

1 green bell pepper, stem and seeds removed, finely diced

¼ cup balsamic vinegar

1½ teaspoons chopped fresh basil

Salt and freshly ground black pepper

2 (7-ounce) packages of shirataki noodles, such as Dukan Diet Shirataki Noodles, prepared according to the directions on page 232.

1. In a large bowl, thoroughly combine the artichoke hearts, alfalfa sprouts, bell pepper, vinegar, and basil. Add salt and pepper to taste.

2. Add the prepared noodles, stir well, cover, and refrigerate for at least 2 hours before serving.

Shirataki Noodles Primavera with Ranch Sauce

MAKES 4 SERVINGS

Preparation time: 10 minutes, plus 2 hours for marinating

Cooking time: 5 minutes

1 head of broccoli, chopped into florets

4 carrots, sliced

1 tomato, quartered

1 red onion, sliced

2 (7-ounce) packages of shirataki noodles, such as Dukan Diet
  Shirataki Noodles, prepared according to the directions on
  page 232.

RANCH SAUCE

½ cup Dukan Mayonnaise (page 331)

2 tablespoons fat-free plain Greek-style yogurt

2 tablespoons fat-free sour cream

½ teaspoon chopped fresh chives

½ teaspoon chopped fresh parsley

½ teaspoon chopped fresh dill

¼ teaspoon powdered garlic

¼ teaspoon powdered onion

Salt and freshly ground black pepper

1. Fill the bottom part of a large steamer halfway with water and bring to a simmer.

2. Place the broccoli, carrots, tomato, and onion in the top part of the steamer, cover, and steam for 5 minutes. Remove vegetables and set aside.

3. To make the sauce, in a large bowl, combine the mayonnaise, yogurt, sour cream, chives, parsley, dill, and the garlic and onion powder. Add salt and pepper to taste.

4. Add the vegetables and the prepared noodles, combine thoroughly, cover, and refrigerate for at least 2 hours before serving.

Note: You will need a large steamer for this recipe.

Garlicky Shrimp and Shirataki Noodle Stir-Fry

MAKES 1 SERVING

Preparation time: 5 minutes

Cooking time: 10 minutes

⅛ teaspoon olive oil

1½ teaspoons finely chopped fresh garlic

1 tablespoon finely chopped shallots or onion

6 ounces shrimp, peeled and deveined

1 tablespoon chopped fresh herbs, such as parsley, sorrel, or basil

Thai hot sauce, such as Sriracha (optional)

1 (7-ounce) package of shirataki noodles, such as Dukan Diet
    Shirataki Noodles, prepared according to the directions on
    page 232.

1. Heat a large, heavy-bottomed skillet over medium heat. Add
   the oil, and wipe out any excess with a paper towel.
2. Add the garlic and shallots and cook, stirring often, for 3 to
   4 minutes.
3. Add the shrimp and cook, stirring often. After 1 minute, add
   the herbs.
4. Continue cooking until the shrimp turn pink, about 3 additional minutes.
5. Add the Sriracha sauce if desired, and serve over the noodles.

Note: Add baby spinach, sliced mushrooms, and diced red and yellow
bell peppers, if you like.

Discover Dukan Diet Shirataki Noodles

Discover Dukan Diet Organic Stevia

—— *Seafood, Fish, and Vegetables* ——

Calamari Provençal

MAKES 4 SERVINGS

Preparation time: 20 minutes

Cooking time: 25 minutes

⅛ teaspoon vegetable oil

1 large onion, finely chopped

3 cups canned, diced low-sodium tomatoes

3 garlic cloves, very finely chopped

1 green bell pepper, seeds removed, diced

1 bouquet garni (make your own by tying together 6 sprigs of fresh parsley, 3 sprigs of fresh thyme, and 3 dried bay leaves)

1 fresh red or green chili pepper, very finely chopped

Salt and freshly ground black pepper

1 pound 2 ounces calamari, cleaned and cut into rings

1. Heat a heavy-bottomed pan over medium heat. Add the oil and wipe out any excess with a paper towel.
2. Add the onion and cook until browned, stirring often, about 5 minutes.
3. Add the tomatoes, garlic, bell pepper, bouquet garni, and chili pepper, plus salt and pepper to taste.
4. Reduce the heat, cover, and cook for 15 minutes.
5. Add the calamari, cover, and cook for an additional 2 minutes.

Mussel Stew with Leeks

MAKES 4 SERVINGS
Preparation time: 30 minutes
Cooking time: 30 minutes

4 pounds mussels, scrubbed clean
2¼ pounds leeks (white parts only), sliced
Salt and freshly ground black pepper
A pinch of grated nutmeg
½ cup White Sauce (page 339)
1 bunch of fresh parsley, very finely chopped
1 bunch of fresh chervil, very finely chopped
1 sprig of fresh tarragon, very finely chopped
Juice of ½ lemon

1. Place the cleaned mussels in a large pot. Discard any that are open or broken, and add 2 cups of water.
2. Cover the pot and cook over high heat until the water comes to a boil.
3. Reduce the heat, and simmer until the mussels open, about 4 to 5 minutes. During cooking, shake the pot so the mussels can cook evenly.
4. Discard any mussels that haven't opened and save the cooking liquid.
5. Remove the mussels from their shells and set them aside.
6. Strain the cooking liquid, pour it into a deep skillet, and bring the liquid to a boil.
7. Add the leeks to the cooking liquid, reduce the heat, cover, and cook for 5 minutes.
8. Remove the lid, add salt and pepper to taste and nutmeg, and cook for an additional 10 minutes.
9. Add the mussels to the leeks. Add the white sauce, parsley, chervil, tarragon, and lemon juice and mix thoroughly.
10. Serve hot.

Baked Mussels

MAKES 4 SERVINGS

Preparation time: 30 minutes

Cooking time: 30 minutes

⅛ teaspoon vegetable oil

1 pound 10 ounces zucchini, sliced

Salt and freshly ground black pepper

2¼ pounds mussels, scrubbed clean

1 bay leaf

2 teaspoons cornstarch

2 teaspoons fat-free sour cream (optional)

8 egg yolks

8 teaspoons fat-free plain Greek-style yogurt

6 tablespoons fat-free cream cheese (optional)

1. Preheat oven to 475°F.
2. Heat a medium, heavy-bottomed skillet over medium heat. Add the oil and wipe out any excess with a paper towel.
3. Add the zucchini, season with salt and pepper to taste, and cook for 10 minutes, stirring often.
4. While the zucchini is cooking, place the cleaned mussels in a large pot. Discard any that are open or broken. Add the bay leaf and 2 cups of water.
5. Once the zucchini is cooked, remove it from the pan and drain.
6. Cover the large pot, and cook the mussels over high heat until the liquid comes to a boil.
7. Reduce the heat to a simmer, and cook until the mussels open, about 4 to 5 minutes. During cooking, shake the pot so the mussels can cook evenly.
8. Discard any mussels that haven't opened and save the cooking liquid.
9. Remove the mussels from their shells and set them aside.
10. Strain the cooking liquid and let it cool.
11. In a saucepan off the heat, mix the cornstarch with 1 cup of the cooled cooking liquid from the mussels and the crème fraîche (if using), and blend until smooth.

12. Heat the mixture over medium heat, add pepper to taste, and whisk until thickened, about 10 minutes.

13. In a medium bowl, mix the egg yolks and yogurt, add the cornstarch mixture, and continue stirring until thoroughly combined.

14. Place the zucchini slices in a 9 × 9-inch baking dish, top with the mussels, and cover with the sauce. Top with dollops of cream cheese (if using).

15. Place the dish in the oven and bake for 5 minutes, then turn the oven up to Broil and broil for an additional 2 minutes.

Seafood and Vegetable Appetizers with Herb Cream Sauce

MAKES 6 SERVINGS
Preparation time: 30 minutes
Cooking time: No cooking required

FOR THE SAUCE
1 cup fat-free plain Greek-style yogurt
3 fresh basil leaves, finely chopped
3 sprigs of fresh tarragon, finely chopped
3 sprigs of fresh parsley, finely chopped
Salt and freshly ground black pepper

1 cucumber, peeled and cut into strips
3 carrots, cut into strips
1 bunch of radishes, sliced
1 fennel bulb, cut into strips
3 stalks of celery sticks, each cut in 3 pieces
7 ounces cooked shrimp, peeled with tails removed
3 surimi (crab sticks), each cut in 2 pieces

1. To make the sauce, in a small bowl, mix together the yogurt, basil, tarragon, and parsley. Add salt and pepper to taste.

2. Serve the sauce as a dip for the vegetables and seafood.

Shrimp-Stuffed Tomatoes

MAKES 2 SERVINGS

Preparation time: 15 minutes

Cooking time: 10 minutes

4 eggs

1 pound 2 ounces tomatoes

Salt and freshly ground black pepper

1¼ pounds shrimp, cooked and shelled, with tails removed

1 teaspoon mustard

1 tablespoon fresh lemon juice

¾ cup fat-free plain Greek-style yogurt

1. Place the eggs in a large pot and cover with cold water. Bring to a boil. Once the water is boiling, reduce to a simmer and cook the eggs for 10 minutes.

2. Remove the eggs from the hot water and help them to cool by running cold water over them. Remove the shells.

3. Cut 2 of the eggs into quarters and set aside. Remove the yolks from the remaining 2 eggs and set them aside in a separate bowl, discarding the whites.

4. Cut the tomatoes in half and scoop out their insides. Discard the seeds, sprinkle the hollowed-out tomatoes with salt to taste, and place on a plate to drain.

5. In a food processor combine the shrimp and the 2 quartered hard-boiled eggs. Pulse until the mixture is finely chopped.

6. Stuff the tomatoes with the shrimp mixture.

7. Crush the 2 remaining yolks with the back of a fork and combine with the mustard, lemon juice, and salt and pepper to taste. Mix in the yogurt and stir until thoroughly combined.

8. When ready to serve, top the stuffed tomatoes with the yogurt sauce.

Stir-Fried Garlic Shrimp and Mushrooms

MAKES 4 SERVINGS

Preparation time: 25 minutes

Cooking time: 7 to 8 minutes

⅛ teaspoon vegetable oil

1 pound shrimp, shelled, tails removed, chopped

2 garlic cloves, chopped

1 pound button mushrooms, thinly sliced

1 pound surimi (crab sticks), cut into cubes

Salt and freshly ground black pepper

1 bunch of fresh parsley, chopped

1. Heat a nonstick frying pan over medium heat. Add oil and wipe out any excess with a paper towel. Add the shrimp and garlic, and cook for 5 minutes, stirring often. Add the mushrooms and cook for 1 additional minute.

2. Add the surimi, season with salt and pepper to taste, stir in the parsley, and serve immediately.

Cucumber Roulades with Shrimp

MAKES 2 SERVINGS

Preparation time: 20 minutes, plus 1 hour for chilling

Cooking time: 10 minutes

2 eggs

4 ounces shrimp, cooked and shelled, chopped

¾ cup fat-free plain Greek-style yogurt

A few drops of Tabasco sauce

Salt and freshly ground black pepper

1 cucumber

¼ cup chopped chives

1. Place the eggs in a large pot and cover with cold water. Bring to a boil. Once the water is boiling, reduce the heat to a simmer and cook the eggs for 10 minutes.

2. Remove the eggs from the hot water and help them to cool by running cold water over them.

3. Peel the eggs, place them in a bowl, and mash them with a fork.

4. Add the shrimp, yogurt, and Tabasco. Season with salt and pepper to taste.

5. Peel the cucumber, cut it in half lengthwise, and scoop out the middle. Stuff each half with the shrimp mixture and sprinkle the chopped chives on top.

6. Place half of the cucumber on top of the other half so there is cucumber on the bottom, filling in the middle, and a cucumber on top.

7. Refrigerate for 1 hour. Slice crosswise, and serve.

Baked Fish with Shrimp and Asparagus

MAKES 4 SERVINGS
Preparation time: 15 minutes
Cooking time: 30 minutes

⅛ teaspoon vegetable oil
14 ounces white fish fillets, such as cod, red snapper,
    or flounder, cut into small pieces
5 ounces shelled shrimp, tails removed
¼ cup fat-free plain Greek-style yogurt
6 spears of fresh asparagus, cut into ½-inch pieces
3 sprigs of fresh parsley
Salt and freshly ground black pepper
4 egg whites

1. Preheat oven to 350°F.

2. Add the oil to a baking dish, using a paper towel to coat it and to wipe out any excess.

3. In a medium bowl, mix together the fish pieces, shrimp, yogurt, asparagus, and parsley, and add salt and pepper to taste.

4. In a medium mixing bowl, beat the egg whites until stiff, then gently fold them into the fish mixture.
5. Transfer this mixture into the prepared dish and bake in the oven for 30 minutes.

Shrimp and Egg Salad

MAKES 2 SERVINGS
Preparation time: 15 minutes
Cooking time: 15 minutes

½ teaspoon olive oil
4 teaspoons cider vinegar
Salt and freshly ground black pepper
1¼ pounds lettuce, such as romaine, red leaf, or butter
3 sprigs of fresh tarragon
7 ounces shrimp, cooked and shelled, with tails removed
4 eggs

1. In a small bowl, whisk together the olive oil and vinegar, and add salt and pepper to taste.
2. In a large bowl, toss the lettuce, tarragon, and shelled shrimp.
3. Place the eggs in a large pot and cover them with cold water. Bring the water to a boil, then reduce it to a simmer and cook the eggs for 5 minutes.
4. Remove the eggs from the hot water and shell them carefully while they are still warm, as the yolks will still be runny.
5. Transfer the salad with the olive oil dressing and top with the warm eggs.

Green Chili Shrimp

MAKES 4 SERVINGS
Preparation time: 10 minutes
Cooking time: 5 minutes

4 tomatoes, stems removed
1 fresh green chili, seeds removed, chopped
2 tablespoons chopped fresh cilantro
Juice of 1 lime
1 garlic clove, crushed
Salt
32 large shrimp

1. Fill a medium pot with water and bring to a boil. Add the tomatoes and poach for 30 seconds. Remove the tomatoes from the pot, peel off the skin, remove the seeds, and dice.
2. In a medium bowl, mix the tomatoes, chili, cilantro, lime juice, and garlic, plus salt to taste, until combined.
3. Fill the bottom part of a large steamer halfway with water and bring to a simmer.
4. Place the shrimp in the top part of the steamer and cook until they turn pink and opaque, about 3 minutes.
5. Mix the shrimp with the tomato mixture and serve warm or chilled.

Note: You will need a large steamer for this recipe.

Asparagus and Seafood Salad

MAKES 2 SERVINGS

Preparation time: 10 minutes

Cooking time: 15 minutes

4 eggs

1 pound asparagus

1 low-sodium vegetable bouillon cube

2 tomatoes, stems and seeds removed, chopped

10 surimi (crab sticks), chopped

1 head of lettuce, such as romaine or red leaf, leaves separated

Vinaigrette Maya (page 330)

1. Place the eggs in a large pot and cover with cold water. Bring the water to a boil. Once the water is boiling, reduce the heat to a simmer, and cook the eggs for 10 minutes.
2. Remove the eggs from the hot water and help them to cool by running cold water over them. Remove the shells and cut each egg in half lengthwise.
3. Peel the asparagus and snap off the woody bottoms at their natural breaking point. Discard the bottoms.
4. Fill a pot with water, add the bouillon cube, and bring the water to a boil. Add the asparagus and blanch for 3 minutes.
5. Remove the asparagus from the pot, drain, and chop into ½-inch pieces.
6. In a bowl, mix the asparagus, tomatoes, chopped surimi, and eggs.
7. Arrange the lettuce leaves in the bottom of a round dish and fill each leaf with an equal amount of the asparagus mixture.
8. Dress the salad with the vinaigrette.

Seafood Casserole

MAKES 3 TO 4 SERVINGS

Preparation time: 10 minutes

Cooking time: 30 minutes

⅛ teaspoon vegetable oil

10 ounces surimi (crab sticks), sliced

8 eggs, beaten

½ cup tomato paste

3 tablespoons fat-free plain Greek-style yogurt

3 sprigs of fresh parsley

Salt and freshly ground black pepper

1. Preheat oven to 325°F.
2. Add the oil to a heatproof casserole, using a paper towel to coat it and to wipe out any excess.
3. In a large bowl, mix the surimi, eggs, tomato paste, yogurt, and parsley, plus salt and pepper to taste, until thoroughly combined.
4. Fill the prepared casserole with the egg mixture, and bake for 30 minutes. Serve hot.

Seafood Terrine

MAKES 2 SERVINGS

Preparation time: 15 minutes

Cooking time: 30 minutes

¼ cup oat bran, such as Dukan Diet Organic Oat Bran

3 tablespoons fat-free plain Greek-style yogurt

3 eggs, beaten

5 ounces mixed seafood, such as cod, shrimp, and scallops, shelled if using shellfish, and chopped

2 tablespoons finely chopped fresh herbs of your choice, such as parsley, sorrel, and basil

Salt and freshly ground black pepper

1. Preheat oven to 350°F. Line a 9-inch-square pan or loaf pan with parchment paper or wax paper.
2. In a large bowl, thoroughly combine the oat bran, yogurt, eggs, seafood, and herbs, along with salt and pepper to taste.
3. Pour the mixture into the prepared pan, and bake for 30 minutes.

Note: As a substitute for sorrel, you may use the same amount of spinach, with the addition of 1 teaspoon of lemon juice.

Note: You will need a 9-in-square pan or loaf pan for this recipe.

Seared Scallops with Sorrel

MAKES 2 SERVINGS
Preparation time: 15 minutes
Cooking time: 10 minutes

8 ounces sea or bay scallops
Salt and freshly ground black pepper
¼ teaspoon oil
12 medium sorrel leaves (see Note)
2 shallots, finely chopped
4 teaspoons fat-free plain Greek-style yogurt

1. If using sea scallops, cut in half to make 2 circles. Season the scallops with salt and pepper to taste.
2. Heat a medium nonstick frying pan over high heat. Add ⅛ teaspoon of the oil and wipe out any excess with a paper towel.
3. Place the scallops in the prepared pan and cook until just browned on each side, about 1 minute per side. Remove from the pan and set aside.
4. Place the sorrel leaves in the same frying pan, reduce the heat to medium, and cook until wilted, stirring often, about 3 minutes.
5. Meanwhile, heat a small, heavy-bottomed pan over medium

heat. Add the remaining ⅛ teaspoon of oil and wipe out any excess with a paper towel.

6. Place the shallots in the small pan and cook until soft, stirring often, about 5 minutes.

7. Once shallots are soft, turn the heat off, and immediately stir in the yogurt.

8. To serve, place a spoonful of sorrel onto each plate, top with scallops, and pour the shallot sauce over them. Serve warm.

Note: As a substitute for sorrel, you may use the same amount of spinach, with the addition of 1 teaspoon of lemon juice.

Scallop and Spinach Bake

MAKES 2 SERVINGS
Preparation time: 30 minutes
Cooking time: 20 minutes

¼ teaspoon vegetable oil
1 pound bay scallops
1 pound fresh spinach, finely chopped
2 egg yolks, beaten
3 tablespoons fat-free plain Greek-style yogurt
1 tablespoon cornstarch
1¼ cups cold low-sodium fish stock
Salt and freshly ground black pepper

1. Preheat oven to 400°F.

2. Add ⅛ teaspoon of the oil to two 1½-cup ramekins and wipe out any excess with a paper towel.

3. Heat a large, heavy-bottomed skillet over medium heat. Add the remaining oil and wipe out any excess with a paper towel.

4. Add the scallops, and cook, stirring continuously, for 2 minutes.

5. Add the spinach to the skillet and cook for 1 additional minute, stirring constantly.

6. Remove the spinach and scallop mixture from the pan and divide it between the two prepared ramekins.

7. In a small saucepan, combine the egg yolks and yogurt.

8. In a small bowl, mix the cornstarch and cold fish stock until thoroughly combined, and add to the pan with the yogurt mixture. Season with salt and pepper to taste.

9. Heat the yogurt mixture over low heat until just warmed through.

10. Pour the sauce over the scallop mixture and bake for 15 minutes. Serve in the ramekin dishes.

Note: You will need two 1½-cup ramekins for this recipe.

Scallop and Grilled Vegetable Salad

MAKES 2 SERVINGS

Preparation time: 10 minutes, plus 1 hour for refrigerating
Cooking time: 25 minutes

Grated zest and juice of 1 lemon
2 tablespoons finely chopped fresh cilantro
Salt and freshly ground black pepper
16 bay scallops
1 eggplant, cut into cubes
2 zucchini, sliced
⅛ teaspoon vegetable oil
¼ cup tomato-based sauce, such as Paprika and Red Pepper
    Sauce (page 341) or Grelette Sauce (page 342)

1. In a small bowl, combine the lemon zest and juice, cilantro, and salt and pepper to taste. Set aside.

2. Fill the bottom part of a large steamer halfway with water and bring to a simmer.

3. Place the scallops in the top part of the steamer, cover, and cook for 3 minutes, then remove and set aside.

4. Place the eggplant and zucchini in the top part of the steamer, cover, and cook for 10 minutes.

5. Heat a heavy-bottomed skillet over medium heat. Add the oil and wipe out any excess with a paper towel.

6. Add the steamed vegetables. Cook, stirring often, for 5 minutes and remove from heat.

7. Add the lemon marinade and stir to thoroughly combine.

8. To serve, spread the tomato-based sauce onto two plates. Top each with half the vegetables and then the scallops. Cover and refrigerate for 1 hour before serving.

Note: You will need a large steamer for this recipe.

Tuna and Caper–Stuffed Tomatoes
MAKES 4 SERVINGS
Preparation time: 20 minutes
Cooking time: 5 minutes

8 tomatoes, with stems removed
Salt and freshly ground black pepper
1 (5-ounce) can tuna packed in water, drained
¾ cup fat-free plain Greek-style yogurt
2 tablespoons capers, drained and rinsed
2 tablespoons very finely chopped fresh chives
1 tablespoon fresh lemon juice
2 tablespoons caviar (trout roe)
1 teaspoon paprika

1. Fill a pot with water and bring it to a boil. Add the tomatoes and poach for 30 seconds. Remove the tomatoes from the pot and peel off the skin.

2. Slice off the tops of the tomatoes and set them aside.

3. Scoop out the insides of the tomatoes, sprinkle some salt inside, and turn them upside down on paper towels to let their juices drain.

4. In a medium bowl, mix together the tuna, yogurt, capers, chives, and lemon juice, plus pepper to taste, until thoroughly combined.

5. Stuff the tomatoes with the tuna mixture, and top with the trout roe and paprika.

6. Replace the tops of the tomatoes before serving.

Crustless Tuna and Tomato Quiche

MAKES 3 SERVINGS
Preparation time: 15 minutes
Cooking time: 30 minutes

2 eggs

4 egg whites

⅛ teaspoon vegetable oil

2 small tomatoes, very thinly sliced

1 (5-ounce) can of tuna packed in water, drained and flaked

2 tablespoons fat-free plain Greek-style yogurt

2 pinches of herbes de Provence (a mix of dried marjoram, thyme, savory, basil, rosemary, sage, and fennel seeds)

Salt and freshly ground black pepper

1. Preheat oven to 350°F.

2. In a small bowl, beat the eggs and the egg whites.

3. Heat a 9-inch nonstick skillet over medium heat. Add the oil and wipe out any excess with a paper towel.

4. Pour in the eggs and cook until set, as though making an omelet.

5. Transfer the omelet in a 9-inch pie plate.

6. In a medium bowl, mix the tomatoes, tuna, yogurt, and herbs, plus salt and pepper to taste, until thoroughly combined.

7. Top the omelet with the vegetable mixture and bake for 25 minutes. Serve warm.

Creamed Tuna

MAKES 2 SERVINGS
Preparation time: 10 minutes
Cooking time: 15 minutes

⅞ cup tuna canned in water, drained and flaked
1 onion, finely chopped
1 garlic clove, finely chopped
10½ ounces zucchini, thinly sliced
3 tablespoons tomato paste
Salt and freshly ground black pepper

1. Heat 2¼ cups of water in a saucepan.
2. Add the tuna, onion, garlic, zucchini, and tomato paste, plus salt and pepper to taste.
3. Reduce the heat, cover, and cook for 15 minutes. Serve warm.

Three-Pepper Tuna

MAKES 3 TO 4 SERVINGS
Preparation time: 20 minutes, plus 2 to 3 hours for marinating
Cooking time: 30 minutes

1 red bell pepper
1 green bell pepper
1 yellow bell pepper
⅛ teaspoon vegetable oil
Juice of 1 to 2 lemons
2 garlic cloves, crushed
1 pound 9 ounces tuna steak
Salt and white pepper

1. Turn oven on to Broil. Place the bell peppers on a baking sheet and broil, turning every few minutes until they are charred on all sides, about 10 minutes.
2. Immediately place the peppers in a bowl and cover with a plate to steam.

3. Once the peppers have cooled, peel off the skin, remove the seeds, and cut into strips.

4. Heat a large, heavy-bottomed skillet over medium heat. Add the oil and wipe out any excess with a paper towel.

5. Add the peppers and cook, stirring often, for 5 minutes.

6. Place the cooked peppers in a medium bowl and mix with the lemon juice and garlic.

7. Fill the bottom part of a large steamer halfway with water and bring the water to a simmer.

8. Season the tuna with salt and white pepper to taste and place in the top part of the steamer. Cover and cook for 10 minutes, then remove from the steamer and let cool.

9. Place the tuna in a shallow dish and pour the bell pepper mixture over it.

10. Cover the dish and place it in the refrigerator for 2 to 3 hours to marinate, turning the tuna over every 30 minutes.

Note: You will need a large steamer for this recipe.

Tuna-Stuffed Cucumber

MAKES 1 SERVING
Preparation time: 15 minutes
Cooking time: No cooking required

1 cucumber
1 (5 ounce) can tuna packed in water, drained and flaked
4 teaspoons Dukan Mayonnaise (page 331)
Salt and freshly ground black pepper

1. Peel the cucumber, cut it in half lengthwise, then cut each piece in half.

2. Scoop out the seeds and some flesh with a spoon.

3. In a medium bowl, mix the tuna and mayonnaise, and season with salt and pepper to taste.

4. Stuff the cucumber boats with the tuna mixture.

Tuna Pizza

MAKES 1 SERVING

Preparation time: 20 minutes

Cooking time: 45 minutes

2 tablespoons oat bran, such as Dukan Diet Organic Oat Bran

1 tablespoon fat-free plain Greek-style yogurt

1½ tablespoons fat-free ricotta

3 eggs, separated

Salt and freshly ground black pepper

¼ teaspoon vegetable oil

1 large onion, finely chopped

1 pound tomatoes, stems and seeds removed, chopped

1 teaspoon mixed fresh or dried herbs such as thyme, oregano, and basil

1 (5-ounce) can tuna packed in water, drained and chopped

2 tablespoons capers, drained and rinsed

3 tablespoons fat-free cream cheese (optional)

1. Preheat oven to 375°F.
2. In a medium bowl, mix the oat bran, yogurt, ricotta, and egg yolks, plus salt and pepper to taste, until thoroughly combined.
3. In a medium mixing bowl, beat the egg whites until stiff and fold them into the oat bran mixture.
4. Heat a medium nonstick frying pan over medium heat. Add ⅛ teaspoon of oil and wipe out any excess with a paper towel.
5. Pour the oat bran mixture into the hot pan and cook until browned on one side, about 3 minutes. Using a spatula, turn the galette over and continue cooking on the other side until browned, about 2 more minutes.
6. Meanwhile, heat an additional nonstick pan over medium heat. Add the remaining oil and wipe out any excess with a paper towel.
7. Add the onion and cook, stirring often, until soft, about 5 minutes.

8. Add the tomatoes and herbs, plus salt and pepper to taste, and simmer for 10 minutes.
9. In a small bowl, mix the tuna, capers, and cream cheese (if using).
10. Spread the tomato mixture over the galette, and top with the tuna mixture.
11. Bake for 25 minutes.

Normandy Cod Fillets

MAKES 2 SERVINGS
Preparation time: 20 minutes
Cooking time: 25 minutes

5 ounces mussels, scrubbed clean
10 ounces skinless cod fillets
1 dried bay leaf
3 sprigs of fresh thyme
1 teaspoon chopped garlic
1 teaspoon tomato paste
4 teaspoons fat-free plain Greek-style yogurt
Salt and freshly ground black pepper

1. Place the cleaned mussels in a pot with a lid, discarding any that are open or broken and that do not close when tapped.
2. Add 2 cups of water, cover the pot, and cook the mussels over high heat until the liquid comes to a boil. Reduce the heat to a simmer, and cook until the mussels open, about 4 to 5 minutes.
3. During cooking, shake the pot so the mussels can cook evenly.
4. Once the mussels have cooked, discard any unopened ones. Remove the rest of the mussels from their shells and reserve. Save ½ cup of the cooking liquid, strain it, and set aside.
5. In a heatproof casserole, place the cod, bay leaf, thyme, garlic, and ½ cup of the cooking liquid from the mussels.

6. Place the casserole over low heat, bring to a simmer, and cook for 10 minutes. Remove the fish to a serving dish and leave the cooking liquid in the casserole.

7. Add the tomato paste, yogurt, and mussels to the casserole, cook for 2 minutes over low heat, and season with salt and pepper to taste. Remove the bay leaf.

8. Pour sauce over the cod fillets when ready to serve.

Sole Ceviche on a Bed of Tomatoes

MAKES 2 SERVINGS
Preparation time: 10 minutes, plus 1 hour for refrigeration
Cooking time: 10 minutes

4 ripe tomatoes
Juice of 1 lemon
Salt and freshly ground black pepper
8 ounces skinless sole fillets, cut into paper-thin strips
1 sprig of fresh mint, very finely chopped
1 sprig of fresh chervil, very finely chopped
1 sprig of fresh parsley, very finely chopped

1. Fill a medium pot with water and bring to a boil. Add the tomatoes and poach for 30 seconds. Remove the tomatoes from the pot, peel off the skin, remove the seeds, and chop the tomatoes finely.

2. In a medium bowl, mix the tomatoes and lemon juice, plus salt and pepper to taste, until thoroughly combined. Spread a bed of the tomatoes on two plates.

3. Lay the strips of fish in a single layer atop the tomato mixture and sprinkle on the herbs and salt and pepper to taste.

4. Cover and refrigerate for 1 hour. Serve cold.

Note: Eating raw fish carries some risk of food-borne illness. Raw fish should not be consumed by the very young, the very old, pregnant women, or anyone with a compromised immune system.

Baked Sole with Tomato Sauce

MAKES 2 SERVINGS
Preparation time: 25 minutes
Cooking time: 30 minutes

⅛ teaspoon vegetable oil

1 pound tomatoes

14 ounces skinless sole fillets, cut into ½-inch pieces

Salt and freshly ground black pepper

1 bunch of fresh chervil, leaves removed and stems discarded

2 tablespoons plus 1 teaspoon fat-free plain Greek-style yogurt

1 sprig of fresh thyme

1 dried bay leaf

1 garlic clove, crushed

1 shallot, chopped

1. Preheat oven to 400°F.
2. Coat two 1-cup ramekins with the oil and wipe out any excess with a paper towel.
3. Fill a medium pot with water and bring to a boil. Add the tomatoes and poach for 30 seconds. Remove the tomatoes from the pot and peel off the skin.
4. In a medium bowl, combine the sole fillets, salt and pepper to taste, chervil, and yogurt. Pour the fish mixture into the prepared ramekin dishes.
5. Place the ramekins into a baking dish large enough to fit them, and fill the baking dish half full with cold water.
6. Place the baking dish in the oven and cook until the mixture is browned on the top, about 20 to 25 minutes.
7. Remove the ramekins from the oven and let rest for 3 minutes before turning contents out onto serving dishes.
8. Meanwhile, in a saucepan, place the tomatoes, thyme, bay leaf, garlic, and shallot, bring to a simmer, and cook for 15 minutes. Remove the bay leaf.
9. To serve, pour tomato sauce over the cooked fish.

Note: You will need two 1-cup ramekins for this recipe.

Quick Fillet of Sole

MAKES 1 SERVING
Preparation time: 10 minutes
Cooking time: 2 minutes

7 ounces skinless sole fillet
1 fresh tomato, stem removed, finely chopped
1 garlic clove, chopped
½ teaspoon capers, drained and rinsed
4 fresh basil leaves, torn

1. Place the sole in a microwave-safe dish.
2. In a small bowl, mix the tomato, garlic, capers, and basil until thoroughly combined.
3. Spread this tomato mixture over the fish, cover, and microwave for 2 minutes on High.

Fillet of Sole with Sorrel

MAKES 2 SERVINGS
Preparation time: 20 minutes, plus 2 hours for marinating
Cooking time: 4 minutes

10 ounces skinless sole fillets, divided into 2 portions
Juice of 2 lemons, divided
10 medium sorrel leaves, chopped (see Note)
⅛ teaspoon vegetable oil
Salt and freshly ground black pepper

1. Place the sole in a shallow nonreactive dish, and sprinkle half the lemon juice and half the sorrel leaves over the fish.
2. Cover and refrigerate for at least 2 hours.
3. Remove the fish from the marinade. Discard the marinade.
4. Heat a medium nonstick skillet over medium heat. Add the oil and wipe out any excess with a paper towel.
5. Add the fish and cook for 2 minutes on each side.

6. To serve, season the fish with the remaining half of the lemon juice, the remaining sorrel leaves, and salt and pepper to taste.

Note: As a substitute for sorrel, you may use the same amount of spinach, with the addition of 1 teaspoon of lemon juice.

Saffron Tilapia

MAKES 2 SERVINGS

Preparation time: 20 minutes

Cooking time: 35 minutes

Salt and freshly ground black pepper
2 leeks (white parts only), thinly sliced
2 carrots, chopped
2 stalks of celery, chopped
1 onion, cut into quarters, each quarter studded with a clove
1 bouquet garni (make your own by tying together 6 sprigs
of fresh parsley, 3 sprigs of fresh thyme, and 3 dried bay
leaves)
5 black peppercorns
A pinch of saffron
Salt and freshly ground black papper.
10 ounces skinless tilapia fillet, divided into 2 portions
1 tablespoon chopped fresh parsley

1. Place 4 cups of water in a medium pot, add a small pinch of salt, and bring to a boil.
2. Add the leeks, carrots, and celery, and cook for 5 minutes.
3. Add the onion, bouquet garni, peppercorns, and saffron. Reduce the heat to a simmer, cover, and cook for 25 minutes.
4. Remove the vegetables from the broth and reserve.
5. Season the broth with salt and pepper to taste, add the tilapia, and poach for 3 minutes.
6. Carefully remove the fish from the broth with a large slotted spoon.

7. When ready to serve, place the fish on a serving plate sur-rounded by the vegetables, top with a ladleful of stock, and garnish with the chopped parsley. Serve hot.

Warm Tilapia and Green Bean Salad

MAKES 2 SERVINGS
Preparation time: 25 minutes
Cooking time: 15 minutes

3 cups low-sodium fish stock
10 ounces skinless tilapia fillet, divided into 2 portions
Salt and freshly ground black pepper
4 ounces green beans
1 tablespoon raspberry vinegar
⅛ teaspoon hazelnut (or other nut) or vegetable oil
1 garlic clove, crushed
1 shallot, very finely chopped

1. Add the fish stock to a medium pot and bring to a boil. Add the tilapia and poach for 3 minutes. Carefully remove the fish with a slotted spoon and set it aside. Discard the fish stock.
2. Meanwhile, fill a medium pot with water, add a small pinch of salt, and bring the water to a boil. Add the beans and blanch for 3 minutes, then remove and run cold water over them. Drain them and place them in a bowl.
3. In a small bowl, combine the vinegar, oil, garlic, and shallot, and season with salt and pepper to taste.
4. Dress the beans with two-thirds of the vinaigrette.
5. To serve, place a pile of the beans on each of two plates, top with the tilapia, and finish with the remaining vinaigrette.

Creole Tilapia

MAKES 2 SERVINGS

Preparation time: 25 minutes, plus 2 hours for refrigeration

Cooking time: 30 minutes

1 garlic clove

1 onion, quartered, each quarter studded with a clove

3 sprigs of fresh thyme

1 carrot

Salt and freshly ground black pepper

8 ounces skinless tilapia fillet

½ (7-gram) envelope of unflavored gelatin (3½ grams)

8 large lettuce leaves, such as romaine or red leaf

1 lime, quartered

6 fresh mint leaves, chopped

1. In a large pot, place 6 cups of water and the garlic, onion, thyme, and carrot, plus salt and pepper to taste. Bring to a boil, then reduce the heat and simmer for 20 minutes.
2. Add the tilapia and poach for 3 minutes. Carefully remove the fish with a slotted spoon, then chop it and set it aside. Strain the cooking liquid and reserve.
3. Place 2¼ cups of the warm stock in a bowl, add the gelatin, stir to dissolve, and let sit for 5 minutes.
4. Mix the chopped fish into the stock and gelatin mixture and pour into two 2-cup ramekins.
5. Cover the ramekins and refrigerate for 2 hours.
6. Make a bed of lettuce on each of two plates.
7. To turn the fish out of the ramekins, place them in a warm water bath, taking care not to let the water run over the tops. Gently run a knife around the inside edge of each ramekin, and ease the fish out onto the lettuce beds.
8. Garnish with the lime quarters and chopped mint.

Note: You will need two 2-cup ramekins for this recipe.

Saffron Cod

MAKES 3 SERVINGS
Preparation time: 15 minutes
Cooking time: 40 minutes

1 pound tomatoes, stems and seeds removed, cut into chunks
2 garlic cloves, crushed
1 leek (white parts only), finely chopped
1 medium onion, chopped
1 fennel bulb, finely chopped
3 sprigs of fresh parsley
1 pinch of saffron
Salt and freshly ground black pepper
21 ounces skinless cod fillet, split into 3 portions

1. In a heatproof casserole, place the tomatoes, garlic, leeks, onion, fennel, parsley, and saffron, plus salt and pepper to taste. Simmer over low heat for 30 minutes.
2. Add the cod and ½ cup of water, and bring to a boil, then immediately reduce the heat to a simmer.
3. Simmer the fish until it is opaque in the center, about 5 minutes for a ½-inch-thick fillet, 10 minutes for a 1-inch-thick fillet.

Baked Cod with Zucchini and Thyme

MAKES 2 SERVINGS
Preparation time: 10 minutes
Cooking time: 30 minutes

⅛ teaspoon vegetable oil
3 medium zucchini, stems removed and sliced
1 garlic clove, crushed
2 teaspoons chopped fresh thyme leaves
Salt and freshly ground black pepper
14 ounces skinless cod fillet, sliced

1. Preheat oven to 375°F.
2. Coat a small baking dish with the vegetable oil, using a paper towel to wipe out any excess.
3. In a medium bowl, season the zucchini slices with the garlic, thyme, and salt and pepper to taste.
4. In a separate bowl, season the fish with salt and pepper to taste.
5. Line the bottom of the prepared baking dish with half of the zucchini, add the fish, and top with the remaining zucchini.
6. Cover with foil and bake for 30 minutes.

Roasted Cod with Zucchini and Tomato

MAKES 4 SERVINGS
Preparation time: 20 minutes
Cooking time: 35 minutes

10 ounces tomatoes
4 medium zucchini, cut into ⅛-inch-thick slices
2 sprigs of fresh thyme
Salt and freshly ground black pepper
28 ounces skinless cod fillet
4 garlic cloves, cut into 3 slices each

1. Preheat oven to 425°F.
2. Fill a medium pot with water and bring to a boil. Add the tomatoes and poach for 30 seconds. Remove the tomatoes from the pot, peel off the skin, and remove the seeds. Chop the tomatoes finely.
3. In a 9 × 13-inch baking dish, place 1 tablespoon of water and add the tomatoes, zucchini, and thyme, plus salt and pepper to taste. Mix together well.
4. Make six incisions in each side of the fish fillet, deep enough to insert the garlic slices. Insert the garlic, and season with salt and pepper to taste.
5. Place the fish in the center of the baking dish, moving the vegetables to the sides.

6. Place the dish in the oven and roast for 30 minutes, stirring the vegetables several times so they cook evenly.
7. To serve, place the fish on a platter with the vegetables and pour the cooking juices over the top.

Curried Cod

MAKES 4 SERVINGS
Preparation time: 20 minutes
Cooking time: 35 minutes

⅛ teaspoon vegetable oil
1 onion, chopped
3 garlic cloves, crushed
4 dried chili peppers, finely chopped
4 mild fresh chili peppers, chopped
1 teaspoon coriander seeds
1 teaspoon ground turmeric
1 teaspoon ground cumin
1 pound 2 ounces tomatoes, stems and seeds removed, chopped
3 tablespoons fresh lemon juice
28 ounces skinless cod fillet, cut into ½-inch slices
Salt and freshly ground black pepper

1. Heat a medium nonstick skillet over medium heat. Add the oil and wipe out any excess with a paper towel.
2. Add the onion, garlic, and the dried and fresh chilies, and cook until the onion is soft, about 5 minutes.
3. Add the coriander, turmeric, and cumin, and cook for an additional 5 minutes.
4. Mix in the tomatoes, ¼ cup water, and the lemon juice.
5. Bring everything to a boil, reduce the heat, cover, and simmer for 15 minutes.
6. Add the fish, season with salt and pepper to taste, and cook for an additional 10 minutes.

Baked Cod with Herbs and Peppers

MAKES 4 SERVINGS

Preparation time: 20 minutes

Cooking time: 20 minutes

1 shallot, finely chopped

1 onion, finely chopped

1 bunch of fresh herbs, finely chopped, such as oregano,
   rosemary, or thyme

28 ounces skinless cod fillet, divided into 4 portions

Salt and freshly ground black pepper to taste

1 red bell pepper, quartered, with seeds removed

4 small fresh chili peppers, halved

Grated zest and juice of 1 lemon

1. Preheat oven to 425°F.
2. Lay out four 8 × 8-inch pieces of aluminum foil.
3. In a small bowl, mix the shallot and onion with the herbs.
4. Place a fillet on each piece of aluminum foil.
5. Season each fillet with salt and pepper to taste. Top with a piece of bell pepper, a thin layer of the herb mixture, and a chili pepper.
6. Pour the lemon juice over the fish and sprinkle the lemon zest on top.
7. Carefully seal the foil parcels, put them on a baking sheet, and bake for 20 minutes.

Baked Cod Provençal

MAKES 4 SERVINGS

Preparation time: 25 minutes

Cooking time: 20 minutes

¼ teaspoon vegetable oil

8 slices of extra-lean ham

8 tomatoes, with stems removed

Salt and freshly ground black pepper

2 onions, thinly sliced

2 garlic cloves, thinly sliced

28 ounces skinless cod fillets, divided into 4 portions

3 fresh basil leaves, chopped

1. Preheat oven to 475°F.
2. Divide the oil among the four 2-cup ramekins. Wipe out the excess with a paper towel.
3. Place one slice of ham into each ramekin.
4. Fill a large pot with water and bring to a boil. Add the tomatoes and poach for 30 seconds.
5. Remove the tomatoes from the pot, peel off the skin, and remove the seeds.
6. Slice the tomatoes and divide them evenly among the ramekins, placing them on top of the ham.
7. Sprinkle salt to taste on the tomatoes and top with the onion and garlic slices.
8. Wrap each portion of cod fillet in a slice of ham and place in a ramekin.
9. Season with salt and pepper to taste and bake for 15 minutes.
10. Remove the ramekins from the oven, add more black pepper to taste, and sprinkle the chopped basil leaves on top.

Note: You will need four 2-cup ramekins for this recipe.

Salmon with Endive

MAKES 1 SERVING
Preparation time: 10 minutes
Cooking time: No cooking required

2 ounces smoked salmon, cut into even strips
1 endive heart, chopped
1 tablespoon chopped fresh dill
Salt and freshly ground black pepper
Juice of 1 lemon
1 tablespoon salmon roe

1. In a medium bowl, combine the smoked salmon, endive, and dill.
2. Season with salt and pepper to taste, and sprinkle with the lemon juice.
3. Top with the salmon roe and serve immediately.

Baked Salmon and Broccoli

MAKES 3 SERVINGS
Preparation time: 15 minutes
Cooking time: 35 minutes

⅛ teaspoon vegetable oil
2 eggs, beaten
2 (6-ounce) cans salmon packed in water, drained
10 ounces broccoli florets
1 cup plus 2 tablespoons fat-free cottage cheese
1 small onion, finely chopped
7 ounces green bell pepper, seeds removed, chopped
Salt and freshly ground black pepper

1. Preheat oven to 350°F.
2. Add oil to 9 × 9-inch nonstick baking dish and wipe out any excess with a paper towel.
3. In a medium bowl, mix the eggs, salmon, broccoli, cottage

cheese, onion, and bell pepper, plus salt and paper to taste, until thoroughly combined.

4. Transfer the mixture to the prepared baking dish, and bake for 35 minutes.

Salmon Rolls

MAKES 8 SERVINGS
Preparation time: 20 minutes
Cooking time: 20 minutes

⅛ teaspoon vegetable oil
8 slices of smoked salmon
2 (14-ounce) cans of hearts of palm
¼ cup fat-free ricotta
½ cup plus 1 tablespoon fat-free plain Greek-style yogurt
2 pinches of herbes de Provence (a mixture of dried marjoram, thyme, savory, basil, rosemary, sage, and fennel seeds)
⅛ teaspoon raspberry vinegar
Salt and freshly ground black pepper

1. Preheat oven to 300°F.
2. Add oil to 9 × 9-inch baking dish and wipe out any excess with a paper towel.
3. Wrap the smoked salmon slices around the hearts of palm.
4. In a medium bowl, mix together the ricotta, yogurt, herbs, and vinegar, plus salt and pepper to taste.
5. Pour half of the ricotta mixture into the prepared baking dish. Place the smoked salmon on top, and pour the rest of the ricotta mixture on top of the salmon.
6. Bake in the oven for 20 minutes.

Salmon with Fennel Salad

MAKES 2 SERVINGS
Preparation time: 20 minutes
Cooking time: No cooking required

Juice of ½ lemon
1¼ cups fat-free plain Greek-style yogurt
Salt and freshly ground black pepper
½ fennel bulb, cut into small chunks
1 small bunch of fresh dill, finely chopped
4 slices of smoked salmon, cut into thin strips
4 lettuce leaves, such as romaine, red leaf, or butter

1. In a small bowl, combine the lemon juice and yogurt. Add salt and pepper to taste.
2. Add the fennel and dill.
3. To serve, divide the salmon slices between two plates. Fill the lettuce leaves with the fennel mixture and place two of them on each plate.

Triple Salmon Bake

MAKES 4 SERVINGS
Preparation time: 20 minutes, plus 2 hours for refrigeration
Cooking time: 10 minutes

4 (4-ounce) salmon steaks
2 low-sodium fish bouillon cubes
2 (7-gram) envelopes of unflavored gelatin
4 sprigs of fresh dill
2 ounces salmon roe
1 slice of smoked salmon, cut into strips
4 cups mesclun mix

1. Place four 2-cup ramekins in the freezer.
2. Fill the bottom part of a large steamer halfway with water and bring the water to a simmer.

3. Place the salmon steaks in the top part of the steamer, cover, and cook for 5 minutes.
4. Take the salmon out of the steamer and remove any bones.
5. In a medium pot, place 1 cup of water and the bouillon cubes. Bring the mixture to a boil, and cook for 5 minutes to dissolve the cubes and reduce the bouillon.
6. Remove the broth from the heat and add the gelatin.
7. Take the ramekins out of the freezer, and fill each with 2 tablespoons of the fish broth mixture.
8. Inside each ramekin, add a sprig of dill, a steamed salmon steak, some of the salmon roe (reserve a little for garnish), and a quarter of the smoked salmon strips.
9. Distribute the remaining fish broth mixture among the 4 ramekins, cover, and refrigerate for 2 hours.
10. To serve, turn the ramekins out onto 4 plates, top each with a little salmon roe, and serve with mesclun.

Note: You will need a large steamer and four 2-cup ramekins for this recipe.

Salmon on a Bed of Leeks

MAKES 2 TO 3 SERVINGS
Preparation time: 15 minutes
Cooking time: 30 minutes

¼ cup chopped shallots
3 leeks (white parts only), finely chopped
Salt and freshly ground black pepper
⅛ teaspoon vegetable oil
1 pound 4 ounces salmon fillets, divided into 4 portions
1 tablespoon chopped fresh dill

1. Place the shallots, leeks, and 3 tablespoons of water in a heavy-bottomed skillet and cook over low heat for 20 minutes.
2. Season with salt and pepper to taste, turn off heat, and cover to keep warm.

3. Heat a nonstick frying pan over medium heat. Add the oil and wipe out any excess with a paper towel. Place the fish in the pan with the skin side down. Cook until the flesh turns light pink. Depending on the thickness of the fillets, this will take 2 to 5 minutes.

4. Flip the salmon and cook for an additional 2 to 5 minutes.

5. To serve, place the leeks on a large serving plate and top with the salmon and chopped dill.

Salmon and Fennel Terrine

MAKES 4 SERVINGS

Preparation time: 40 minutes

Cooking time: 1 hour

1¼ pounds fennel, diced

1 pound skinless salmon fillet

2 egg whites

Salt and freshly ground black pepper

¾ cup fat-free plain Greek-style yogurt

A pinch of curry powder

1 tablespoon very finely chopped fresh dill

1. Preheat oven to 350°F.

2. Line a 9-inch loaf pan with parchment paper.

3. Fill the bottom part of a large steamer halfway with water and bring to a simmer.

4. Place the fennel in the top part of steamer, cover, and cook for 10 minutes.

5. Drain the fennel, place it in a blender, and process until puréed, about 1 minute.

6. Reserve 3 tablespoons of the fennel purée and set the rest aside.

7. Cut two-thirds of the salmon into big chunks and the other third into thin strips.

8. Put the 3 tablespoons of the fennel purée back into the

blender and add the salmon chunks, 1 egg white, and salt and pepper to taste. Blend until puréed, about 1 minute.

9. In a medium bowl, combine the remainder of the fennel, the yogurt, salt and pepper to taste, curry powder, and the remaining egg white.

10. Into the prepared loaf pan, place half of the salmon purée and top with half of the chopped dill.

11. On top of the dill, place one-third of the fennel purée, then one-half of the salmon strips.

12. Follow with another third of the fennel purée, then the remaining salmon strips. End with the remaining fennel purée.

13. Top with the remaining chopped dill and a layer of the remaining salmon purée.

14. Cover the loaf pan and place it into a bigger baking dish and fill that dish halfway with cold water.

15. Place the larger dish in the oven, and bake for 45 minutes.

Note: You will need a 9-inch loaf pan and a large steamer for this recipe.

Salmon with Salsa Verde on a Bed of Cherry Tomatoes

MAKES 2 SERVINGS
Preparation time: 15 minutes
Cooking time: 30 minutes

10 ounces cherry tomatoes, halved
10 ounces skinless salmon fillets, divided into 2 portions
1 teaspoon of chopped fresh herbs, singly or mixed, such as dill, chives, and basil
¼ cup salsa verde (a Mexican sauce made from green tomatoes and chilies, available in jars or cans)

1. Preheat oven to 400°F.
2. Cut 2 pieces of 9 × 9-inch parchment paper. Place half the cherry tomatoes, salmon fillets, herbs, and salsa verde in the center of each piece.

3. Fold one half of the parchment over the other and twist on both ends. Tie up the ends of the parchment paper with butcher's twine.

4. Place the parcels on a baking sheet, and bake for 30 minutes.

Salmon with Fennel and Leeks

MAKES 4 SERVINGS
Preparation time: 15 minutes
Cooking time: 35 minutes

1 egg
Salt
4 leeks (white parts only), cut lengthways
2 fennel bulbs, cut into quarters
4 onions, cut into quarters, each quarter studded with 4 cloves
1 bouquet garni (make your own by tying together 6 sprigs
    of fresh parsley, 3 sprigs of fresh thyme, and 3 dried bay
    leaves)
4 (5-ounce) salmon steaks

1. Place the egg in a small pot and cover with cold water. Bring to a boil. Once the water is boiling, reduce the heat to a simmer, and cook the egg for 10 minutes.

2. Remove the egg from the hot water and let it cool by running cold water over it. Peel the egg and chop.

3. Fill a large pot with water, add a small pinch of salt, and bring to a boil.

4. Add the leeks, fennel, onions, and bouquet garni. Reduce the heat to a simmer and cook for 10 minutes.

5. Add the salmon steaks and continue cooking for another 5 minutes.

6. Remove the fish and vegetables from the poaching liquid, top with the chopped egg, and serve.

Salmon and Bresaola Salad

MAKES 4 SERVINGS
Preparation time: 20 minutes
Cooking time: 3 minutes

1 teaspoon olive oil
3 tablespoons balsamic vinegar
Salt and freshly ground black pepper
4 cups mixed salad greens
4 ounces thinly sliced bresaola or cooked turkey bacon
1 pound 9 ounces skinless salmon, cut into large cubes
3 pink peppercorns, crushed
3 sprigs of fresh chervil, chopped

1. In a small bowl, combine the oil, vinegar, and salt and pepper to taste.
2. Divide the salad greens equally among 4 plates.
3. Place the bresaola slices on top of the salad.
4. Heat a heavy-bottomed skillet over medium heat, and cook the salmon cubes, stirring constantly until cooked on all sides, about 3 minutes.
5. Place the salmon atop the salad and dress with the balsamic dressing.
6. Top with the pink peppercorns and chervil.

Smoked Salmon Mousse

MAKES 2 SERVINGS

Preparation time: 15 minutes, plus 2 to 3 hours for refrigeration

Cooking time: No cooking required

5 ounces smoked salmon

1 cup plus 1 tablespoon fat-free plain Greek-style yogurt

½ (7-gram) envelope (about 1 teaspoon) of unflavored gelatin

1 teaspoon tomato paste

Juice of 1 lemon

A pinch of paprika

2 egg whites

¼ teaspoon vegetable oil

4 stalks of celery

1. In a blender, process the smoked salmon and yogurt until fully puréed, about 1 minute.
2. In a small bowl, combine 2 tablespoons of water with the gelatin. Let sit for 5 minutes.
3. Add the gelatin mixture, tomato paste, lemon juice, and paprika to the salmon mixture.
4. Transfer the salmon mixture to a large bowl.
5. In a mixing bowl, beat egg whites until stiff.
6. Fold the egg whites into the salmon mixture.
7. Divide the oil among the two 1-cup ramekins. Use a paper towel to coat and wipe out the excess.
8. Spoon the mixture into the ramekins, cover, and refrigerate for 2 to 3 hours.
9. Serve with the celery sticks.

Note: You will need two 1-cup ramekins for this recipe.

Smoked Salmon and Cucumber Terrine

MAKES 2 SERVINGS

Preparation time: 30 minutes, plus 1 hour for refrigeration

Cooking time: No cooking required

1 cucumber, peeled, cut in half lengthwise, and seeds removed

Salt and freshly ground black pepper

½ bunch of fresh chives, finely chopped

7 ounces smoked salmon, cut into very thin slices

¾ cup plus 1 tablespoon fat-free cottage cheese

1. Cut the cucumber into small cubes, place in a bowl, sprinkle with a little salt, cover, and refrigerate for 30 minutes.
2. In a medium bowl, combine the chives, salmon, and pepper to taste.
3. Drain the cottage cheese of as much liquid as possible.
4. Drain the diced cucumber and rinse it several times, then dry on kitchen towels.
5. Add the cucumber to the salmon and chive mixture.
6. Beat the drained cottage cheese with a whisk and stir it into the salmon mixture.
7. Season with salt and pepper to taste, cover, and refrigerate for at least 1 hour before serving.

Baked Salmon and Vegetable Parcels

MAKES 4 SERVINGS

Preparation time: 20 minutes

Cooking time: 30 minutes

1 small zucchini, stem removed

2 tomatoes, stems removed

¼ pound button mushrooms, thinly sliced

4 (5-ounce) salmon steaks

1 lemon, cut into quarters

Salt and freshly ground black pepper

2 teaspoons pink peppercorns

1. Preheat oven to 425°F.
2. Prepare four 9 × 9-inch squares of parchment paper.
3. Thinly slice the zucchini, without removing its skin.
4. Bring a pot of water to a boil. Add the tomatoes and poach for 30 seconds. Remove the tomatoes from the pot, peel off the skin, remove the seeds, and cut into quarters.
5. In a medium bowl, place the tomatoes, the sliced zucchini, and the mushrooms.
6. Place each salmon steak on a piece of parchment paper.
7. Top each salmon steak with the vegetables and a lemon quarter.
8. Season with salt and pepper to taste and top with pink peppercorns.
9. Fold each piece of parchment paper into a parcel and seal with butcher's twine. Place the parcels on a baking sheet and bake for 25 minutes.

Minted Salmon

MAKES 4 SERVINGS

Preparation time: 20 minutes, plus refrigeration overnight
Cooking time: 30 minutes

1 pound skinless salmon fillet
⅛ teaspoon vegetable oil
1 large zucchini, stem removed and thinly sliced lengthwise
1 (7-gram) envelope of unflavored gelatin
1 slice of smoked salmon, diced
1 tablespoon fat-free plain Greek-style yogurt
3 tablespoons chopped fresh mint
Salt and freshly ground black pepper

1. Preheat oven to 375°F.
2. Wrap the salmon fillet in foil and bake it for 30 minutes.
3. Unwrap the salmon, let it cool, then roughly chop it and place the pieces in a large bowl.

4. Heat a medium-size heavy-bottomed skillet over medium heat. Add the oil and wipe out any excess with a paper towel.

5. Add the zucchini and cook, stirring often, until browned, about 5 minutes.

6. In a small saucepan, combine the gelatin and 2 tablespoons of water. Let sit for 5 minutes, then heat over low heat until dissolved.

7. Mix the gelatin, smoked salmon, yogurt, and mint with the cooked salmon.

8. Season with salt and pepper to taste.

9. Line four 2-cup ramekins with the zucchini slices and add the salmon mixture.

10. Cover and refrigerate overnight or for 12 hours,

11. Remove the ramekins from the refrigerator and let sit for 30 minutes before serving.

Note: You will need four 2-cup ramekins for this recipe.

Crab and Tomato–Stuffed Flounder

MAKES 4 SERVINGS
Preparation time: 15 minutes
Cooking time: 30 minutes

⅛ teaspoon vegetable oil
1 small onion, chopped
1 stalk of celery, chopped
1 tablespoon finely chopped fresh parsley
4 ounces white crabmeat
1 egg, beaten
Salt and freshly ground black pepper
1 pound 12 ounces flounder, cut into 8 slices
1 cup low-sodium tomato juice

1. Preheat oven to 425°F.

2. Coat a baking dish with the oil, using a paper towel to wipe out any excess.

3. In a medium bowl, mix the onion, celery, parsley, crabmeat, and egg until thoroughly combined. Season with salt and pepper to taste.

4. Place 4 slices of fish in the prepared dish.

5. Spread the crab mixture over each of the 4 fish slices and top with the other 4 slices of fish.

6. Pour the tomato juice over the fish and bake for 30 minutes.

Indian-Style Sea Bass and Shrimp

MAKES 4 SERVINGS

Preparation time: 15 minutes, plus 1 hour for marinating

Cooking time: 25 minutes

1 tablespoon garam masala

1¼ cups fat-free plain Greek-style yogurt

14 ounces sea bass fillet, cut into chunks

7 ounces large shrimp, shelled

Salt and freshly ground black pepper

¼ teaspoon vegetable oil

2 shallots, very finely chopped

5 carrots, cut into very thin strips

7 ounces fennel, cut into very thin strips

2 tablespoons low-sodium vegetable stock

1 teaspoon cornstarch

1 cup watercress

1 tablespoon lemon juice

1. In a small bowl, combine the garam masala and ¾ cup of the yogurt.

2. In a mixing bowl, season the sea bass and shrimp with salt to taste, then coat with the yogurt mixture.

3. Cover and refrigerate for at least 1 hour.

4. Drain the fish and shrimp and place on a paper towel.

5. Heat a medium, heavy-bottomed skillet over high heat. Add ⅛ teaspoon of the oil and wipe out any excess with a paper towel.

6. Add the fish and shrimp and cook, stirring often, for 3 minutes.

7. Remove the pan from the heat and cover to keep warm.

8. Heat a nonstick pan over medium heat. Add the remaining oil and wipe out any excess with a paper towel.

9. Add the shallots and cook, stirring continuously, for 3 minutes. Add the carrots and fennel and cook for an additional 3 minutes.

10. Add the vegetable stock, reduce the heat, cover, and cook until the vegetables are tender, about 5 minutes.

11. In a small bowl, add the remaining ½ cup of the yogurt, the cornstarch, and 1 teaspoon of cold water. Mix until thoroughly combined.

12. Whisking continuously, pour this yogurt mixture into the pan with the vegetables and bring to a simmer.

13. Add the cooked fish and shrimp and warm through.

14. To serve, garnish with watercress, lemon juice, and salt and pepper to taste.

Seafood Fondue

MAKES 4 SERVINGS

Preparation time: 25 minutes

Cooking time: 10 minutes

1¼ pounds mixed vegetables, such as cabbage, carrots,
    mushrooms, celery, and tomatoes, cut into bite-size pieces
4 cups low-sodium fish stock
Salt and freshly ground black pepper
3 sprigs of fresh chervil
14 ounces fish, such as monkfish, cod, or red snapper, cubed
4 ounces calamari, sliced
12 large shrimp, peeled
1 lemon, sliced

1. Fill a pot with water and bring it to a boil. Add the vegetables and poach for 2 minutes.

2. Remove the vegetables from the water, drain, and divide among 4 plates.

3. Place the stock in a pot, bring it to a boil, season with salt and pepper to taste, and add the chervil.

4. Divide the seafood among the 4 plates, placing it atop the vegetables. Top with the lemon slices.

5. Place the stock in a lit fondue pot, and bring it to the dining table.

6. Dip the vegetables and fish into the stock until cooked, about 2 to 3 minutes. Make sure that the stock remains at a simmer while cooking the fish and vegetables.

Note: You will need a fondue set for this recipe.

Spinach and Smoked Fish Salad

MAKES 4 SERVINGS
Preparation time: 5 minutes
Cooking time: 2 minutes

1 pound 9 ounces baby spinach
10 ounces smoked fish, such as salmon or trout,
    cut into ¾-inch strips
2 teaspoons mustard
1 teaspoon white wine vinegar
⅛ teaspoon hazelnut or vegetable oil
Salt and freshly ground black pepper

1. Wash and pat dry the young spinach leaves and arrange on individual plates.

2. Heat a medium, heavy-bottomed skillet over medium heat. Add ⅛ teaspoon of the oil and wipe out any excess with a paper towel. Add the fish, and cook, stirring constantly, for 2 minutes.

3. Remove the fish from the skillet and place atop the spinach.

4. In a small bowl, combine the mustard, vinegar, and oil. Add salt and pepper to taste.

5. Drizzle the dressing over the fish and spinach.

Baked Fish Parcels

MAKES 4 SERVINGS

Preparation time: 20 minutes

Cooking time: 10 minutes

28 ounces of lean fish fillet, such as cod, red snapper, or
flounder, divided into 4 portions

2 onions, finely chopped

2 tomatoes, stems removed, finely chopped

2 carrots, finely chopped

1 green bell pepper, with seeds removed, finely chopped

2 stalks of celery, finely chopped

2 sprigs of fresh parsley, finely chopped

Salt and freshly ground black pepper

1. Preheat oven to 475°F.

2. Place each piece of fish on a 9 × 9-inch sheet of parchment paper.

3. Top each piece of fish with the onions, tomatoes, carrots, bell pepper, celery, parsley, and salt and pepper to taste.

4. Fold each piece of parchment paper into a parcel and seal with butcher's twine. Place the parcels on a baking sheet.

5. Turn the oven down to 400°F, and bake the parcels for 10 minutes.

Fish Stew

MAKES 2 SERVINGS

Preparation time: 20 minutes

Cooking time: 30 minutes

⅛ teaspoon vegetable oil

1 pound fish, such as monkfish or cod, cut into chunks

¼ pound button mushrooms, finely chopped

9 ounces mussels, scrubbed clean

1 cup low-sodium fish stock

Juice of ½ lemon

2 tablespoons fat-free plain Greek-style yogurt

1 egg yolk

Salt and freshly ground black pepper

1. Heat a medium, heavy-bottomed skillet over medium heat. Coat with the oil and wipe out any excess with a paper towel.
2. Place the fish and mushrooms in the pan, and cook, stirring often, until golden brown, about 5 minutes.
3. Discard any mussels that are open or broken.
4. Add the remaining mussels and the fish stock to the same skillet and cook for 15 minutes.
5. Drain the fish, reserving the cooking liquid.
6. Discard any unopened mussels.
7. Shell the cooked mussels and set them aside with the fish. Keep warm.
8. Return the cooking liquid to a small pan, reduce the liquid, and strain it. Return the strained liquid to the pan.
9. Stir in the lemon juice, then whisk in the yogurt and egg yolk. Cook over low heat, without allowing the sauce to boil, for 5 minutes.
10. Season with salt and pepper to taste.
11. Pour the sauce over the fish and serve.

Fish and Chive Terrine

MAKES 3 TO 4 SERVINGS

Preparation time: 40 minutes, plus overnight refrigeration

Cooking time: 1 hour

Salt and freshly ground black pepper

10 ounces spinach

7 ounces carrots

14 ounces red snapper fillet, cut into chunks

4 egg whites

⅔ cup plus 2 tablespoons fat-free plain Greek-style yogurt

10 ounces skinless salmon fillet, cut into thin strips

Juice of 1 lemon

1 tablespoon chopped fresh chives or fresh tarragon

1. Bring a pot of lightly salted water to a boil.
2. Add the spinach, cook for 2 minutes, and drain.
3. In a blender, process the spinach for 1 minute.
4. Place the spinach in a strainer over a bowl, cover, and refrigerate overnight.
5. Preheat oven to 350°F.
6. Line a 9-inch loaf pan with parchment paper.
7. Fill the bottom part of a large steamer halfway with water and bring to a simmer. Place the carrots in the top part of the steamer, cover and cook for 10 minutes.
8. In a blender, process the carrots until puréed, about 1 minute. Remove the carrot purée from the blender and reserve.
9. In a clean blender, place the red snapper, egg whites, 2 tablespoons of the yogurt, and salt and pepper to taste. Process until puréed, about 1 minute.
10. Divide the fish mixture among three bowls.
11. Stir the puréed carrots into one bowl, the puréed spinach into the second bowl, and leave the last bowl as is.
12. In the prepared loaf pan, layer each of the fish mixtures, placing a layer of salmon strips between each layer of puréed fish.

13. Bake the terrine for 45 minutes.

14. Meanwhile, in a small bowl, thoroughly combine the remaining ⅔ cup of yogurt with the lemon juice and herbs, plus salt and pepper to taste. Serve the sauce with the terrine.

Note: You will need a 9-inch loaf pan and a large steamer for this recipe.

Spinach and Fish Terrine

MAKES 4 SERVINGS
Preparation time: 15 minutes
Cooking time: 40 minutes

⅛ teaspoon vegetable oil

2¼ cups low-sodium fish stock

28 ounces white fish fillets, such as cod or red snapper, cut into chunks

1 pound frozen spinach, thawed, with excess water squeezed out

Salt and freshly ground black pepper

2 eggs, separated

1. Preheat oven to 425°F.
2. Add the oil to a 9-inch loaf pan, using a paper towel to coat it and to wipe out any excess.
3. In a medium nonstick pan, bring the stock to a boil. Add the fish, reduce the heat, cover, and cook for 5 minutes.
4. Remove the fish from the pan and drain.
5. In a blender, process the spinach, fish, salt and pepper to taste, and the egg yolks until puréed, about 1 minute.
6. Transfer the fish mixture to a large bowl.
7. In a medium mixing bowl, beat the egg whites until stiff.
8. Fold the egg whites into the fish mixture.
9. Fill the prepared loaf pan with the fish mixture.
10. Place the loaf pan inside a larger baking dish, and fill the larger dish halfway with cold water.

11. Place the baking dish in the oven and bake the terrine for 30 minutes. Serve hot or cold from the loaf pan.

Note: You will need a 9-inch loaf pan for this recipe.

Discover Dukan Diet Organic Oat Bran

--------------------- *Vegetables* ---------------------

Asparagus with a Mousseline Sauce

MAKES 2 SERVINGS
Preparation time: 20 minutes
Cooking time: 10 minutes

1¼ pounds asparagus
1 low-sodium vegetable bouillon cube
1 tablespoon cornstarch
1¼ cups fat-free milk
2 eggs, separated
Salt and freshly ground black pepper
Juice of 2 lemons

1. Peel the asparagus and snap off the woody bottoms of the spears at their natural breaking point.
2. Fill a pot with water, add the bouillon cube, and bring to a boil.
3. Add the asparagus and cook until just tender, about 3 minutes. Drain thoroughly.
4. In a medium bowl, whisk together the cornstarch and milk. Transfer to a small saucepan and heat over low heat.
5. Add the egg yolks to the saucepan and cook for an additional 2 minutes, taking care not to boil the sauce. Season with salt and pepper to taste.

6. Add the lemon juice, remove the sauce from the heat, and transfer to a medium-size bowl.

7. In a small mixing bowl, beat the egg whites until stiff, then fold them into the sauce.

8. Pour the sauce over the asparagus and serve warm.

Eggplant Chicken Terrine

MAKES 4 SERVINGS

Preparation time: 25 minutes, plus 30 minutes
for the eggplant juices to drain
Cooking time: 1 hour 10 minutes

Salt

2 eggplants (about 1 pound total), sliced ½ inch thick

⅛ teaspoon vegetable oil

8 ounces cooked chicken or turkey, cut into small cubes

3 stalks of celery, chopped

3 sprigs of fresh parsley, chopped

1 garlic clove, chopped

3 tomatoes, sliced

1. Sprinkle salt over the eggplant slices, place in a colander, and let sit for 30 minutes to drain any juices.

2. Preheat oven to 350°F.

3. Add ⅛ teaspoon of the oil to a 9-inch loaf pan or ovenproof earthenware dish and wipe out any excess with a paper towel.

4. Heat a medium, heavy-bottomed or cast-iron skillet over medium heat. Add the oil and wipe out any excess with a paper towel.

5. Add the chicken and cook until browned, about 5 minutes.

6. Remove the chicken, but leave the juices in the skillet.

7. Add the celery to the skillet and cook, stirring often, until browned, about 5 minutes. Remove and mix with the cooked chicken.

8. In the prepared baking dish, arrange half the eggplant slices

into a layer, then add the chicken mixture, parsley, garlic, and tomato. Top with a layer of the remaining eggplant slices.

9. Bake for 1 hour.

Note: You will need a 9-inch loaf pan or ovenproof earthenware dish for this recipe.

Eggplant Provençal

MAKES 1 SERVING

Preparation time: 15 minutes

Cooking time: 45 minutes

1 medium onion, thinly sliced
1 eggplant (about 4 ounces), peeled and cut into cubes
1 tomato, chopped
1 garlic clove, chopped
2 sprigs of fresh thyme
1 tablespoon chopped fresh basil
Salt and freshly ground black pepper

1. Heat a medium nonstick pan over medium heat, add 2 tablespoons of water and the onion, and cook until the onion is translucent, about 5 minutes.
2. Add the eggplant to the pan and cook until browned, about 5 minutes.
3. Add the tomato, garlic, thyme, and basil to the mixture, and season with salt and pepper to taste.
4. Reduce the heat, cover, and simmer for 30 minutes.

Indian-Style Eggplant

MAKES 2 SERVINGS
Preparation time: 20 minutes
Cooking time: 20 minutes

3 ounces tomato, cut into small pieces
Salt and freshly ground black pepper
1 tablespoon herbes de Provence (a mix of dried marjoram,
   thyme, savory, basil, rosemary, sage, and fennel seeds)
A pinch of curry powder
A pinch of paprika
A pinch of ground coriander
½ pound eggplant, thinly sliced
½ red bell pepper, stems and seeds removed, very thinly sliced

1. Preheat oven to 425°F.
2. Add the oil to a 7 × 7-inch nonstick baking dish and wipe out the excess with a paper towel.
3. Place the tomatoes in a nonstick frying pan and cook over low heat. Season with salt and pepper to taste.
4. Add the herbes de Provence, curry powder, paprika, and coriander.
5. Fill a pot with water, bring to a boil. Add the eggplant and bell pepper and blanch for 2 minutes. Remove the eggplant and pepper, put in a colander, and run cold water over them. Drain.
6. In the prepared baking dish, layer the eggplant, then top with the bell peppers.
7. Pour the tomato sauce over the vegetables and bake for 10 minutes.

Garlic- and Parsley-Stuffed Eggplant

MAKES 2 SERVINGS
Preparation time: 15 minutes
Cooking time: 35 minutes

2 eggplants, about 9 ounces each
1 garlic clove, chopped
2 sprigs of fresh parsley, chopped
Salt and freshly ground black pepper

1. Preheat oven to 375°F.
2. Remove the stems from the eggplants and halve lengthwise.
3. Scoop out the flesh, chop it, and transfer to a large bowl. Add the garlic and parsley, and salt and pepper to taste.
4. Stuff the eggplant halves with the eggplant and garlic mixture.
5. Wrap each eggplant half in a sheet of aluminum foil and bake on a baking sheet for about 35 minutes.

Eggplant with Cilantro and Tomato

MAKES 4 SERVINGS
Preparation time: 30 minutes
Cooking time: 45 minutes

5 large eggplants (about 2 pounds total)
Salt and freshly ground black pepper
⅛ teaspoon vegetable oil
5 tomatoes, sliced
¼ cup finely chopped onion
1 teaspoon chili powder
2½ teaspoons very finely chopped fresh cilantro

1. Preheat oven to 400°F.
2. Wrap 3 of the eggplants in aluminum foil and bake for 30 minutes.
3. Remove the eggplants from the oven, and wait 5 minutes for

them to cool. When they have cooled, hold each from the bottom, peel off the skin, and chop the flesh.

4. Cut the 2 remaining eggplants in half lengthwise.

5. Fill a large pot with water, add a large pinch of salt, and bring to a boil. Add the raw eggplants and cook for 10 minutes.

6. Heat a medium, heavy-bottomed skillet and add oil, wiping out any excess with a paper towel. Place the chopped, previously baked eggplant, and the tomatoes, onion, and chili powder. Season with salt and pepper to taste and cook over medium heat, stirring occasionally for 5 minutes.

7. Scoop the flesh out of the two halved eggplants that you cooked in the boiling water, leaving ½ inch of flesh around the edges.

8. Fill the hollowed-out eggplant halves with the tomato mixture and sprinkle the cilantro on top.

9. Serve hot or cold.

Eggplant Dip

MAKES 4 SERVINGS
Preparation time: 30 minutes
Cooking time: 15 minutes, plus refrigeration time

6 eggplants (about 1 pound 5 ounces total)
2 garlic cloves, crushed
Juice of 1 lemon
1 tablespoon cider vinegar
Salt and freshly ground black pepper
1 teaspoon olive oil (optional)

1. Preheat oven to 425°F.

2. Place the eggplants on a baking sheet, and bake for about 15 minutes until their skins crackle, turning them so they cook on all sides.

3. Remove the eggplants from the oven, and wait 5 minutes for them to cool. Then, holding each from the bottom, peel off the skin.

4. Place the peeled eggplants in a medium bowl and crush the flesh thoroughly with a fork.

5. Add the garlic, lemon juice, and vinegar, and season with salt and pepper to taste.

6. If using olive oil, whisk it into the mixture very slowly, a drop at a time.

7. Refrigerate the dip and serve very cold.

Eggplant Salad

MAKES 2 SERVINGS

Preparation time: 15 minutes, plus 1 hour for refrigeration
Cooking time: 20 minutes

Salt and freshly ground black pepper
2 eggplants, peeled and cut into large cubes
1 teaspoon cider vinegar
1 teaspoon olive oil
1 garlic clove, crushed
4 scallions, finely chopped
1 shallot, very finely chopped
2 sprigs of fresh parsley, chopped

1. Fill a pot with water, add a large pinch of salt, and bring to a boil. Add the eggplants and cook for 5 minutes.

2. Reduce the heat to a simmer and cook for an additional 15 minutes. Remove the eggplants, drain, cool, and crush the flesh with a fork.

3. In a medium bowl, combine the vinegar, oil, garlic, scallions, and shallot.

4. Add the eggplant and mix until thoroughly combined.

5. Cover and refrigerate until cold, at least 1 hour.

6. When ready to serve, garnish with parsley and season with salt and pepper to taste. Serve cold.

Eggplant Strips Provençal

MAKES 2 TO 3 SERVINGS
Preparation time: 20 minutes
Cooking time: 45 minutes

⅛ teaspoon vegetable oil
1 pound 4 ounces eggplant, peeled and cut into long
⅛-inch strips
2 onions, finely chopped
2¼ pounds tomatoes
2 garlic cloves, crushed
Salt and freshly ground black pepper

1. Heat a small heatproof casserole over medium heat. Add the oil to the casserole, using a paper towel to coat it and to wipe out any excess.
2. Add the eggplant and cook until brown, about 5 minutes. Remove the eggplant from the heat and reserve in a medium bowl.
3. Place the onions in the casserole and cook until brown, about 3 minutes.
4. Fill a large pot with water and bring to a boil. Add the tomatoes and poach for 30 seconds. Remove the tomatoes from the pot, peel off the skin, remove the seeds, and chop.
5. Add the tomatoes and garlic to the casserole. Season with salt and pepper to taste.
6. Reduce the heat to low, cover, and cook for 20 minutes.
7. In a blender, process the tomato and onion mixture until puréed, about 1 minute.
8. Return the tomato mixture to the casserole.
9. Add the eggplant strips, cover, and cook over low heat for 15 minutes.
10. Season with salt and pepper to taste. Serve warm.

Eggplant Mousse

MAKES 2 SERVINGS

Preparation time: 40 minutes, plus 6 hours for refrigeration

Cooking time: 25 minutes

1 pound eggplant

2 red bell peppers

2½ tablespoons unflavored gelatin

2 tablespoons sherry vinegar

2 garlic cloves, crushed

1¼ cups fat-free plain Greek-style yogurt

Salt and freshly ground black pepper

1. Preheat oven to 400°F.
2. Place the eggplant and bell peppers on a baking sheet and bake, turning, until skin is blistered on all sides, about 20 minutes.
3. Immediately upon removing the peppers from the oven, place them in a bowl and cover with a plate to steam.
4. In a small saucepan, mix the gelatin and the vinegar until thoroughly combined. Let sit for 5 minutes.
5. Warm the gelatin mixture over low heat, stirring continuously and taking care not to let the mixture boil.
6. Peel off the skin from the bell peppers and remove the seeds and stems.
7. Cut the eggplant in half and scoop out the flesh with a spoon.
8. In a blender, process the garlic, eggplant flesh, and bell peppers until puréed, about 1 minute.
9. Add the gelatin mixture and yogurt to the eggplant mixture in the blender, and season with salt and pepper to taste. Process until thoroughly mixed, about 10 seconds.
10. Pour the eggplant mixture into a small loaf pan, cover, and refrigerate for 6 hours. Serve cold.

Note: You will need a small loaf pan for this recipe.

Swiss Chard with Tofu

MAKES 4 SERVINGS

Preparation time: 20 minutes

Cooking time: 25 minutes

1 pound (1 large bunch) Swiss chard

14 ounces spinach

⅛ teaspoon vegetable oil

½ onion, finely chopped

8 ounces firm tofu, cut into small cubes

1 teaspoon low-sodium soy sauce

Salt and freshly ground black pepper

1 teaspoon very finely chopped fresh mint

1. Wash the chard and the spinach, drain, pat dry, and chop fine.
2. Heat a medium nonstick skillet over medium heat. Add the oil and wipe out any excess with a paper towel.
3. Add the onion and cook until golden brown, about 3 minutes.
4. Add the spinach and chard to the pan, reduce the heat, cover, and cook for 10 minutes.
5. Meanwhile, in a heavy-bottomed or cast-iron skillet, cook the tofu and the soy sauce over low heat for 5 minutes.
6. Season the tofu with salt and pepper to taste and continue cooking for an additional 5 minutes.
7. Serve the hot vegetables with the tofu, and garnish with the chopped mint.

Stuffed Mushrooms

MAKES 6 SERVINGS
Preparation time: 20 minutes
Cooking time: 35 minutes

24 button mushrooms
Salt and freshly ground black pepper
4 ounces zucchini, finely chopped
⅛ teaspoon vegetable oil
2 shallots, chopped
1 garlic clove, chopped
6 ounces extra-lean ham, cut into strips
1 red chili (mild or hot), very finely chopped
A pinch of oat bran, such as Dukan Diet Organic Oat Bran
2 egg yolks
2 tablespoons very finely chopped herbs, singly or mixed, such
   as parsley, basil, chervil, and chives
6 fresh mint leaves, finely chopped
12 fresh chives

1. Preheat oven to 425°F.
2. Clean the mushrooms, then cut the mushroom tops from their stems.
3. In a baking dish, place the mushroom tops, rounded side up, in a single layer.
4. Bake the mushroom tops in the oven for 5 minutes, then remove from the oven and let sit.
5. Chop the mushroom stems and place in a small bowl.
6. Fill a pot with water, add a large pinch of salt, and bring to a boil. Add the zucchini and cook for 2 minutes. Drain.
7. Heat a large, heavy-bottomed or cast-iron skillet over medium heat. Add the oil and wipe out any excess with a paper towel.
8. Add the shallots, garlic, and 1 tablespoon of water to the skillet. Cook until browned, stirring often, about 5 minutes.
9. Add the zucchini, ham, chili, and mushroom stalks and cook, stirring often, until all the moisture has evaporated, about 10 minutes.

10. Remove the mixture from heat and transfer to a medium bowl. Add the oat bran, egg yolks, chopped herbs, and mint.
11. Season with salt and pepper to taste.
12. Fill 12 of the baked mushrooms with the stuffing mixture, then cover them with the remaining 12 mushrooms. Tie them together, using 1 chive each as though it were a string.
13. Place the mushrooms on a baking sheet and bake in the oven for 10 minutes.

Mushrooms à la Grecque

MAKES 2 SERVINGS
Preparation time: 20 minutes
Cooking time: 15 minutes

5 teaspoons lemon juice
2 dried bay leaves
1¼ teaspoons coriander seeds
1 teaspoon freshly ground black pepper
Salt
1½ pounds button mushrooms, chopped
4 teaspoons chopped fresh flat-leaf parsley

1. In a medium saucepan, place 2¼ cups water and the lemon juice, bay leaves, 1 teaspoon of the coriander seeds, the pepper, and a pinch of salt to taste.
2. Bring the water to a boil, cover, and simmer for 10 minutes.
3. Add the mushrooms, return to a boil, and cook for 2 minutes. Turn off the heat.
4. Add the parsley and combine thoroughly.
5. Leave the mushrooms in the saucepan until cold.
6. Drain the mushrooms, reserving the cooking juices from the pan. Remove the bay leaf. Place the drained mushrooms on a serving dish, pour the cooking juices over them, and garnish with remaining ¼ teaspoon coriander seeds.

Cooked Tomato Salsa

MAKES 2 SERVINGS

Preparation time: 20 minutes

Cooking time: 8 minutes, plus 10 minutes for cooling

4 ripe tomatoes

1 red (or white) onion, cut into 8 pieces

2 garlic cloves, crushed

Salt

5 jalapeños

1 tablespoon lemon juice

3 sprigs of fresh cilantro

1. Bring a pot of water to a boil. Add the tomatoes and poach for 30 seconds. Remove the tomatoes from the pot and drain, peel off the skin, remove the seeds, and chop roughly.
2. Place the chopped tomatoes in a food processor. Add the onion, garlic, and a pinch of salt.
3. Cut the jalapeños in half and scoop out the seeds. Either discard the seeds or keep them, depending on how spicy you want your salsa to be.
4. Chop the jalapeños roughly and add them to the food processor, with seeds (if using).
5. Process the sauce until smooth, about 1 minute.
6. Pour the sauce into a saucepan and warm it over medium heat until a pink froth has formed at the top, about 6 to 8 minutes.
7. Remove the pan from the heat and leave to cool for at least 10 minutes.
8. Add the lemon juice and cilantro.

Paprika Tomato Crisps

MAKES 4 SERVINGS
Preparation time: 10 minutes
Cooking time: 2 hours

10 firm and round tomatoes
1 teaspoon mild paprika

1. Preheat oven to 325°F.
2. Cut the tomatoes into ⅛-inch-thick slices.
3. Place the tomatoes on a baking sheet lined with parchment paper and sprinkle with paprika.
4. Bake for 2 hours, until the slices are dry and crisp.
5. Store the tomatoes in an airtight container in a dry place.

Teriyaki Cabbage

MAKES 2 SERVINGS
Preparation time: 25 minutes
Cooking time: 5 minutes

2 tablespoons low-sodium soy sauce
1 tablespoon sugar-free teriyaki sauce
1 garlic clove, crushed
1 teaspoon peeled and grated ginger
Salt and freshly ground black pepper
⅛ teaspoon vegetable oil
1 pound white cabbage, thinly sliced
1 onion, thinly sliced
3 sprigs of fresh thyme

1. In a small bowl, mix the soy sauce, teriyaki sauce, garlic, and ginger, plus pepper to taste, until thoroughly combined. Let sit for at least 5 minutes.
2. Heat a nonstick pan over high heat. Add the oil and wipe out any excess with a paper towel.

3. Add the cabbage, onion, thyme, and salt to taste and cook, stirring often, for 3 minutes.

4. Add the soy sauce mixture to the pan and continue cooking until the liquid has almost completely evaporated. Remove from the heat and serve warm or chilled.

Steamed Cauliflower

MAKES 2 SERVINGS
Preparation time: 10 minutes
Cooking time: 15 minutes

2 eggs
14 ounces cauliflower, cut into florets, stems discarded
Juice of 1 lemon
2 teaspoons chopped fresh parsley
A pinch of ground cumin
Salt and freshly ground black pepper

1. Place the eggs in a large pot and cover with cold water. Bring to a boil. Once the water is boiling, reduce the heat to a simmer and cook the eggs for 10 minutes.

2. Remove the eggs from the hot water and let them cool by running cold water over them. Remove the shells and chop the eggs.

3. Fill the bottom part of a large steamer halfway with water and bring to a simmer.

4. Place the cauliflower in the top part of the steamer, cover, and steam for 5 minutes.

5. Place the cauliflower in a dish and cover with the chopped hard-boiled eggs.

6. Season with the lemon juice, parsley, cumin, and salt and pepper to taste.

Note: You will need a large steamer for this recipe.

Saffron Cream of Cauliflower

MAKES 4 SERVINGS

Preparation time: 20 minutes

Cooking time: 30 minutes

Salt and freshly ground black pepper

1 pound cauliflower, cut into florets, stems discarded

2½ cups fat-free milk

2 garlic cloves

A pinch of ground nutmeg

A pinch of saffron

1 small bunch of fresh chervil, leaves removed and reserved,
  stems discarded

1. Fill a pot with water, add a large pinch of salt, bring to a boil, and blanch the cauliflower for 5 minutes.
2. Drain and refresh the cauliflower by running cold water over it, then drain again.
3. In a medium pot, bring the milk to a boil, then add the cauliflower and garlic.
4. Reduce the heat, cover, and simmer for 20 minutes.
5. Pour the cauliflower mixture into a food processor and process until smooth, about 1 minute.
6. Pour the mixture back into the saucepan and add the nutmeg and saffron.
7. Cook, uncovered, over low heat for 5 minutes without a lid.
8. To serve, pour into a soup tureen, season with salt and pepper to taste, and garnish with the chervil. Serve warm.

Leek Terrine with a Tomato Herb Sauce

MAKES 6 SERVINGS

Preparation time: 30 minutes, plus 3 hours for refrigeration

Cooking time: 20 minutes

4 pounds 8 ounces young leeks or the white parts of leeks

Salt and freshly ground black pepper

4 tomatoes

1 tablespoon wine vinegar

2 tablespoons very finely chopped fresh herbs, singly or mixed, such as chives, thyme, and oregano

1. Line a 9-inch loaf pan with plastic wrap and make a few holes in the wrap so that water can drain.
2. Clean the leeks by trimming the root, about ¼ inch from the white base, and removing and discarding any ragged, coarse outer leaves. Rinse under cold water to remove all dirt and sand.
3. Drain the leeks on paper towels, then cut them lengthwise to fit the length of your loaf pan.
4. Fill a large pot with water and add a large pinch of salt. Bring to a boil.
5. Using butcher's twine, tie the leeks together in small bunches, add to the pot, and blanch for 15 minutes.
6. Drain the leek bunches in a colander and squeeze them to get rid of as much of the cooking water as possible.
7. Arrange the leek bunches in the prepared loaf pan and press down on them firmly.
8. Chill the leeks in the loaf pan for 3 hours; every 30 minutes drain the water that sinks to the bottom of the pan.
9. Meanwhile, fill a large pot with water and bring to a boil. Add the tomatoes and poach for 30 seconds.
10. Remove the tomatoes from the pot, cool, drain, peel off the skins, and remove the seeds.
11. In a food processor, process the tomatoes with the vinegar and herbs until smooth.
12. Season the tomato mixture with salt and pepper to taste.

13. Turn the contents of the loaf pan out onto a large serving dish. Season the top with salt and pepper to taste and serve with the tomato sauce.

Note: You will need a 9-inch loaf pan for this recipe.

Baked Vegetables Provençal

MAKES 6 SERVINGS
Preparation time: 10 minutes
Cooking time: 55 minutes

5 tomatoes, sliced
2 eggplants, peeled and sliced
1 zucchini, sliced
4 red bell peppers, stems and seeds removed, sliced
2 green bell peppers, stems and seeds removed, sliced
8 garlic cloves, unpeeled
A pinch of very finely chopped fresh thyme
A pinch of very finely chopped fresh savory or oregano
5 fresh basil leaves, very finely chopped
Salt and freshly ground black pepper

1. Preheat oven to 425°F.
2. In a large baking dish, arrange the tomatoes, eggplant, and zucchini slices around the edges of the dish, then place the red and green bell peppers and the garlic in the center.
3. Top with the thyme, savory, and basil leaves, and season with salt and pepper to taste.
4. Bake for 30 minutes. Pour 1 cup of water into the pan, without mixing, and continue baking for an additional 25 minutes.
5. Remove the pan from the oven. Squeeze the garlic cloves out of their skin, then chop or mince them before stirring them with the vegetables.

Garden Terrine

MAKES 4 SERVINGS
Preparation time: 15 minutes
Cooking time: 40 minutes

⅛ teaspoon vegetable oil
3 leeks (white and green parts), cleaned
Salt and freshly ground black pepper
2 pounds carrots, grated
5 eggs, beaten
½ cup fat-free plain Greek-style yogurt
4 ounces extra-lean ham, chopped

1. Preheat oven to 375°F.
2. Add oil to a 9-inch loaf pan and wipe out excess with a paper towel.
3. Clean the leeks by trimming the root, about ¼ inch from the white base, and removing and discarding any ragged, coarse outer leaves. Slice them lengthwise. Rinse under cold water to remove all dirt and sand. Drain them on paper towels.
4. Fill a large pot with water, add a large pinch of salt, and bring to a boil. Add the leeks and cook for 20 minutes.
5. Drain the leeks thoroughly and squeeze to remove the excess water.
6. In a large bowl, mix the carrots, leeks, eggs, and yogurt, plus salt and pepper to taste, until thoroughly combined.
7. Stir the ham into the vegetable mixture and pour the mixture into the prepared loaf pan.
8. Cover the loaf pan with aluminum foil and bake for about 20 minutes until golden brown.

Note: You will need a 9-inch loaf pan for this recipe.

Spring Herb Loaf

MAKES 2 SERVINGS

Preparation time: 10 minutes

Cooking time: 30 minutes

⅛ teaspoon vegetable oil

2¼ cups fat-free cottage cheese

1 tablespoon fat-free milk

2 eggs

1 tablespoon fresh sorrel, very finely chopped (see Note)

1 tablespoon fresh basil, very finely chopped

1 tablespoon fresh dandelion leaves, very finely chopped
     (if not available, substitute radicchio)

A pinch of ground cinnamon

Salt and freshly ground black pepper

1. Preheat oven to 350°F.
2. Add the oil to a nonstick 9-inch loaf pan, using a paper towel to coat the pan and to wipe off the excess.
3. Drain the cottage cheese thoroughly.
4. In a medium bowl, beat the cottage cheese, milk, and eggs until as smooth as possible.
5. Add the sorrel, basil, dandelion, cinnamon, and salt and pepper to taste.
6. Pour the batter into the prepared loaf pan and bake for 30 minutes. The loaf can be served either warm or hot.

Note: As a substitute for sorrel, you may use the same amount of spinach, with the addition of 1 teaspoon of lemon juice.

Note: You will need a 9-inch loaf pan for this recipe.

Zucchini Croquettes

MAKES 1 SERVING

Preparation time: 15 minutes, plus 1 hour for the zucchini to marinate

Cooking time: 7 minutes per batch

2 zucchini, grated
Salt and freshly ground black pepper
1 egg
¼ cup cornstarch
⅛ teaspoon vegetable oil

1. Place the grated zucchini in a medium bowl and toss with 1 tablespoon of salt. Let sit for 1 hour.
2. Drain the zucchini thoroughly. Add the egg, plus salt and pepper to taste.
3. Stir in the cornstarch until thoroughly combined, then form the mixture into 6 small balls.
4. Heat a large, heavy-bottomed skillet over medium heat. Add the oil and wipe out any excess with a paper towel.
5. Add the zucchini balls and cook, turning to brown evenly on all sides, about 7 minutes. Remove the balls from heat and serve warm.

Zucchini or Eggplant Purée

MAKES 1 SERVING

Preparation time: 10 minutes, plus 1 hour for refrigeration

Cooking time: 20 minutes

1 tomato
1 medium zucchini or eggplant (about 4 ounces)
1 teaspoon herbes de Provence (a mix of dried marjoram, thyme, savory, basil, rosemary, sage, and fennel seeds)
1 garlic clove, chopped
Salt and freshly ground black pepper

1. Fill a pot with water and bring to a boil. Add the tomato and poach for 30 seconds. Remove the tomato from the pot, drain, peel off the skin, and remove the seeds.
2. Cut the tomato and zucchini or eggplant into approximately equal cubes.
3. Fill the bottom part of a large steamer halfway with water and bring to a simmer.
4. Place the tomatoes and zucchini in the top part of the steamer, cover, and steam for 15 minutes. Remove the vegetables from steamer.
5. In a blender, process the tomatoes and zucchini until smooth. Add the herbes de Provence and garlic, and season with salt and pepper to taste.
6. Cover and refrigerate for at least 1 hour. Serve cold.

Note: You will need a large steamer for this recipe.

Zucchini Peasant-Style

MAKES 2 SERVINGS
Preparation time: 10 minutes
Cooking time: 20 minutes

⅛ teaspoon vegetable oil
9 ounces zucchini, thinly sliced
½ cup fat-free plain Greek-style yogurt
1 teaspoon herbes de Provence (a mix of dried marjoram, thyme, savory, basil, rosemary, sage, and fennel seeds)
Salt and freshly ground black pepper
3 sprigs of fresh parsley, chopped

1. Preheat oven to 425°F.
2. Add the oil to a 7 × 7-inch ovenproof dish and wipe out the excess with a paper towel.
3. Fill the bottom part of a large steamer halfway with water and bring to a simmer.

4. Place the sliced zucchini in the top part of the steamer, cover, and steam until just tender, about 5 minutes.
5. In a medium bowl, mix the yogurt and herbes de Provence, plus salt and pepper to taste, until thoroughly combined.
6. Transfer the zucchini to the prepared baking dish and cover it with the yogurt sauce.
7. Bake for 10 minutes. When ready to serve, top with the chopped parsley.

Note: You will need a large steamer for this recipe.

Zucchini with Tomato Sauce

MAKES 2 SERVINGS
Preparation time: 10 minutes
Cooking time: 35 minutes

⅛ teaspoon vegetable oil
2 zucchini, cut into cubes
4 tomatoes
1 teaspoon herbes de Provence (a mix of dried marjoram, thyme, savory, basil, rosemary, sage, and fennel seeds)
1 garlic clove, crushed
Salt and freshly ground black pepper

1. Add oil to a casserole and wipe out any excess with a paper towel.
2. Place the cubed zucchini in the casserole.
3. Fill a medium pot with water and bring to a boil. Add the tomatoes and poach for 30 seconds. Remove the tomatoes from the pot, peel off the skin, remove the seeds, and chop.
4. Add the chopped tomatoes to the zucchini and mix in the herbes de Provence and garlic.
5. Cover the casserole and cook over low heat for 30 minutes.
6. Season with salt and pepper to taste before serving.

Zucchini with Moroccan Spices

MAKES 2 SERVINGS

Preparation time: 10 minutes

Cooking time: 40 minutes

⅛ teaspoon vegetable oil

2 garlic cloves, crushed

1 teaspoon ground cumin

1 teaspoon ground coriander

1 teaspoon garam masala

1 low-sodium chicken bouillon cube

2 tablespoons tomato purée

4 zucchini, cut into chunks

Juice of 1 lemon

1 bunch of fresh cilantro, leaves removed and stems discarded

1. Heat a heavy-bottomed or a cast-iron skillet over medium heat. Add the oil and wipe out any excess with a paper towel.
2. Add the garlic, cumin, coriander, and garam masala, and cook, stirring continuously, for 3 minutes.
3. Add 2¼ cups of water, the bouillon cube, tomato purée, and zucchini. Reduce the heat and cook for 35 minutes.
4. To serve, drizzle with the lemon juice and top with cilantro.

Tricolor Spinach

MAKES 2 SERVINGS
Preparation time: 10 minutes
Cooking time: 20 minutes

14 ounces frozen spinach
3 tomatoes, chopped
2 yellow bell peppers, stems and seeds removed, finely sliced
3 sprigs of fresh thyme
1 bay leaf
Salt and freshly ground black pepper

1. Fill a medium pot with water and bring to a boil. Add the spinach, return to a boil, and cook for 3 minutes. Remove the spinach from the pot, drain thoroughly, squeeze out excess water, and set aside.
2. Place the tomatoes, bell peppers, thyme, bay leaf, and 1 cup of water into a pot and season with salt and pepper to taste.
3. Cover the pot and cook over low heat for 10 minutes.
4. Add the spinach, and heat thoroughly, about 5 additional minutes. Remove the bay leaf. Serve hot.

Cucumber Mousse

MAKES 2 SERVINGS
Preparation time: 1 hour 25 minutes, plus 12 hours for refrigeration
Cooking time: 5 minutes

2 cucumbers, peeled and sliced
Salt and freshly ground black pepper
½ cup fat-free milk
1 (7-gram) envelope of unflavored gelatin
1¾ cups fat-free plain Greek-style yogurt
Grated zest and juice of 1 lemon
1 onion, chopped
3 sprigs of fresh parsley, very finely chopped
3 sprigs of fresh tarragon, very finely chopped

1. Line a 9-inch nonstick loaf pan with plastic wrap.
2. Place the cucumbers in a small bowl and toss with salt. Let sit for 1 hour, then rinse under cold water and wipe dry.
3. Place the milk in a saucepan and warm over low heat. Add the gelatin and stir until thoroughly dissolved.
4. In a food processor, process the cucumber slices until smooth.
5. Add the yogurt, gelatin-milk mixture, the lemon zest and lemon juice, the onion, parsley, and tarragon to the puréed cucumber. Season with salt and pepper to taste, and process until thoroughly combined, about 30 seconds.
6. Pour the mixture into the prepared loaf pan, cover, and refrigerate for 12 hours. To serve, remove the mousse from the pan and slice.

Note: You will need a loaf pan for this recipe.

Curried Cucumber

MAKES 4 SERVINGS
Preparation time: 20 minutes
Cooking time: 25 minutes

2 medium cucumbers
1 small red or green chili, chopped with or without the seeds,
    depending on taste
1 teaspoon curry powder
4 small tomatoes, quartered
½ cup fat-free milk
1 teaspoon cornstarch
Salt

1. Halve the cucumbers lengthwise, then cut the halves into ½-inch chunks.
2. Heat a nonstick saucepan, add the chili (with seeds, if using), and the curry powder. Cook for 2 minutes, stirring continuously.

3. Add the cucumbers to the pan and cook over low heat for an additional 10 minutes, stirring often.
4. Add the tomatoes and cook for 10 more minutes.
5. In a small bowl, mix the milk and cornstarch until thoroughly combined. Pour over the vegetables.
6. Cook for 1 to 2 minutes, stirring constantly, until the sauce thickens. Add salt to taste. Serve hot.

Tzatziki

MAKES 1 SERVING

Preparation time: 15 minutes, plus 2 hours for refrigeration
Cooking time: No cooking required

½ cucumber, peeled, seeds removed, and finely chopped
Sea salt
1 garlic clove, very finely chopped
¾ cup fat-free plain Greek-style yogurt

1. Place the cucumber in a bowl and sprinkle with a generous pinch of sea salt. Mix and leave the cucumber to sit for 15 minutes, until the juices drain out.
2. Drain the cucumber, and place in a small bowl. Mix in the garlic and yogurt.
3. Cover and refrigerate for at least 2 hours. Serve cold.

Red and Yellow Pepper Mousse

MAKES 4 SERVINGS
Preparation time: 25 minutes
Cooking time: 15 minutes

1 yellow bell pepper
1 red bell pepper
2 teaspoons zero-calorie sweetener suited for cooking and
    baking, such as Splenda
Salt and freshly ground black pepper
5 ounces extra-lean ham
¾ cup plus 1 tablespoon fat-free plain Greek-style yogurt
3 sprigs of fresh parsley, finely chopped

1. Heat oven to Broil. Place the bell peppers on a baking sheet and cook, turning often until charred all over, about 15 minutes.
2. Immediately place the peppers in a bowl and cover with a plate to steam.
3. When the peppers are cool, peel away the skin, remove the seeds, and cut the peppers into slices lengthwise.
4. Put the peppers in a saucepan, cover with cold water, add the sweetener, and season with salt and pepper to taste.
5. Bring the water to a boil and cook for 10 minutes.
6. Drain the peppers, separate four pieces, and dice. Set aside and reserve for garnish.
7. In a food processor, process the bell peppers with the ham until puréed, about 1 minute.
8. Place the purée in a saucepan and cook over low heat for 5 minutes. Pour into a bowl and leave to cool.
9. Before serving, stir the yogurt into the pepper purée and garnish with the diced pepper and chopped parsley.

Parsley Salad

MAKES 2 SERVINGS
Preparation time: 10 minutes
Cooking time: No cooking required

1 large bunch of fresh flat-leaf parsley, leaves removed and
 stems discarded
1 medium onion, finely chopped
Juice of 1 lemon
Salt

1. In a medium bowl, combine the parsley, onion, and lemon
 juice. Season with salt to taste and mix well.
2. Cover and refrigerate. Serve cold.

Note: This salad is an ideal accompaniment for grilled meats.

Shepherd's Salad

MAKES 2 SERVINGS
Preparation time: 15 minutes
Cooking time: No cooking required

4 tomatoes, cut into small chunks
2 small cucumbers, peeled and cut into small chunks
2 onions, thinly sliced
2 bell peppers, stems and seeds removed, chopped
A few fresh mint leaves, finely chopped
3 sprigs of fresh flat-leaf parsley, finely chopped
Juice of ½ lemon
¼ teaspoon olive oil
Salt and freshly ground black pepper

1. In a medium bowl, combine the tomatoes, cucumbers,
 onions, bell peppers, mint, and parsley.
2. Season with the lemon juice, oil, and salt and pepper to taste.
 Serve cold.

Garden Party Cocktail

MAKES 1 SERVING
Preparation time: 10 minutes
Cooking time: 5 minutes

1 medium tomato
1 small carrot
1 small stalk of celery, peeled
Juice of 1 lemon

1. Fill a pot with water and bring to a boil. Place the tomato in the pot and poach for 30 seconds. Drain, peel off the skin, and remove the seeds.
2. Place the tomato, carrot, celery, lemon juice, and ¼ cup water in a juice extractor and juice.
3. Serve the juice very cold.

Note: You will need a juice extractor for this recipe.

Vitality Cocktail

MAKES 2 SERVINGS
Preparation time: 15 minutes
Cooking time: No cooking required

4 medium carrots, cut into small pieces
4 ounces celery root, peeled and cut into small pieces
1 tablespoon finely chopped fresh dill
½ teaspoon salt

1. In a food processor, process the carrots, celery root, dill, salt, with 1¾ cups water until smooth.
2. Serve the juice very cold.

Dukan Goddess Smoothie

MAKES 1 SERVING
Preparation time: 5 minutes
Cooking time: No cooking time required

1 to 2 cups Swiss chard, washed and trimmed
5 baby carrots or 2 regular carrots, coarsely chopped
    (2 beets can be substituted for carrots)
1 tablespoon diced fresh ginger
¼ teaspoon stevia, such as Dukan Diet Organic Stevia
½ cup water
1 to 2 cups ice

Place all ingredients in a blender and process until liquified, about 1 minute. Pour into a glass and drink immediately.

Note: You can add 1 tablespoon Goji berries, a teaspoon of Dukan Diet Organic Cocoa Powder, or a teaspoon of chia or flax seed.

 Desserts

Chocolate Cream

MAKES 4 SERVINGS
Preparation time: 5 minutes, plus 3 hours 15 minutes for cooling
and refrigeration
Cooking time: 25 minutes

1¾ cups fat-free milk
1½ teaspoons ground cinnamon
½ teaspoon vanilla extract
4 teaspoons low-fat cocoa powder, such as Dukan Diet Organic
    Cocoa Powder
3 tablespoons zero-calorie sweetener suited for cooking and
    baking, such as Splenda
4 eggs

1. Preheat oven to 400°F.
2. Place the milk, cinnamon, and vanilla in a saucepan and bring to a boil.
3. Add the cocoa powder and sweetener. Let cool.
4. Place eggs in a medium bowl, beat the eggs, and gradually stir in the milk mixture until thoroughly combined.
5. Pour the mixture from the medium bowl into four 1-cup ramekins.
6. Place the ramekins in a larger baking dish and fill the dish halfway with cold water.
7. Place the large baking dish in the oven and bake until set, about 20 minutes.
8. Remove the ramekins from the oven and let cool for 15 minutes.
9. Cover and refrigerate for at least 3 hours. Serve cold.

Note: You will need four 1-cup ramekins for this recipe.

Cinnamon Cream

MAKES 4 SERVINGS

Preparation time: 5 minutes, plus refrigeration
Cooking time: 10 minutes

1 egg
1 tablespoon cornstarch
2¼ cups cold fat-free milk
½ teaspoon vanilla extract
¼ teaspoon cinnamon
1 teaspoon rum (optional)
2 tablespoons zero-calorie sweetener suited for cooking and baking, such as Splenda
1 egg white

1. In a medium bowl, whisk together the whole egg and cornstarch until thoroughly combined. Add ½ cup of the cold milk.

2. Pour the remaining 1¾ cups of milk into a small saucepan and bring to a boil.

3. Add the hot milk to the cornstarch mixture, whisking continuously. Pour the mixture back into the saucepan.

4. Warm the saucepan over gentle heat, stirring continuously with a wooden spoon.

5. As soon as the mixture starts to boil, remove it from the heat and pour it into a very cold shallow bowl.

6. Add the vanilla, cinnamon, rum (if using), and the sweetener. Mix thoroughly.

7. In a mixing bowl, beat the egg white until stiff. Gently fold it into the warm cream mixture.

8. Cover and refrigerate for at least 3 hours. Serve cold.

Chocolate Pudding

MAKES 4 SERVINGS
Preparation time: 15 minutes, plus refrigeration
Cooking time: 5 minutes

3½ cups cold fat-free milk
3 tablespoons zero-calorie sweetener suited for cooking and baking, such as Splenda
2 tablespoons cornstarch
4 teaspoons low-fat cocoa powder, such as Dukan Diet Organic Cocoa Powder

1. Place 3 cups of the cold milk in a saucepan and bring to a boil.

2. Place the remaining ½ cup of cold milk and the sweetener, cornstarch, and cocoa powder into a cocktail shaker. Shake until mixed thoroughly.

3. Once the milk boils, pour the mixture from the cocktail shaker into the saucepan, stirring continuously.

4. Slowly bring this mixture back to a boil over low heat.

5. Just as the mixture starts to boil pour it into four 1-cup ramekins. Cover and refrigerate at least 3 hours. Serve cold.

Note: You will need a cocktail shaker and four 1-cup ramekins for this recipe.

Flourless Chocolate Cakes

MAKES 2 SERVINGS
Preparation time: 15 minutes
Cooking time: 10 to 15 minutes

⅛ teaspoon vegetable oil

3 large eggs, separated

1 tablespoon zero-calorie sweetener suited for cooking and baking, such as Splenda

2 teaspoons low-fat cocoa powder, such as Dukan Diet Organic Cocoa Powder

1 pinch of ground nutmeg

1. Preheat oven to 350°F.
2. Divide the oil between two 1-cup ramekins. Use a paper towel to coat and remove the excess.
3. In a medium bowl, beat the egg yolks with the sweetener and cocoa powder.
4. In a small mixing bowl, beat the egg whites until stiff.
5. Gently fold the egg whites into the chocolate mixture, add the nutmeg, and pour the mixture into the prepared ramekins.
6. Bake for 10 to 15 minutes.

Note: You will need two 1-cup ramekins for this recipe.

Chocolate Coffee Meringues

MAKES 12 MERINGUES
Preparation time: 10 minutes
Cooking time: 20 minutes

3 egg whites
2 teaspoons low-fat cocoa powder, such as Dukan Diet Organic
   Cocoa Powder
3 tablespoons zero-calorie sweetener suited for cooking and
   baking, such as Splenda
2 teaspoons very strong coffee, cooled

1. Preheat oven to 300°F.
2. Line a baking sheet with parchment paper.
3. In a mixing bowl, beat the egg whites until very stiff.
4. In a small bowl, combine the cocoa powder and the sweetener,
   then fold into the stiff egg whites until thoroughly combined.
5. Add the coffee and continue stirring for about 30 seconds.
6. Drop spoonfuls of the mixture into 12 small mounds on the
   baking sheet. Bake for 20 minutes.

Dukan Ice Cream

MAKES 4 SERVINGS
Preparation time: 15 minutes, plus 2 hours for freezing
Cooking time: No cooking required

½ cup fat-free plain Greek-style yogurt
¼ cup fat-free ricotta
3 egg yolks
1 tablespoon fat-free sour cream (optional)
3 tablespoons zero-calorie sweetener suited for cooking and
   baking, such as Splenda
Flavoring of your choice (coffee, vanilla, lemon zest, cinnamon,
   or low-fat cocoa powder, such as Dukan Diet Organic Cocoa
   Powder), to taste
2 egg whites

1. In a medium bowl, vigorously beat the yogurt, ricotta, egg yolks, crème fraîche (if using), sweetener, and flavoring of your choice for 2 minutes, until thoroughly combined.
2. In a small mixing bowl, beat the egg whites until stiff, then gently fold them into the yogurt mixture.
3. Pour the mixture into an ice tray and freeze until firm, about 2 hours, depending on your freezer.

Note: Raw or undercooked eggs should not be consumed by the very young, the very old, pregnant women, or anyone with a compromised immune system.

Iced Cocoa Soufflé

MAKES 4 SERVINGS

Preparation time: 10 minutes, plus 3 hours for freezing
Cooking time: No cooking required

1 cup fat-free plain Greek-style yogurt
¼ cup low-fat cocoa powder, such as Dukan Diet Organic Cocoa Powder
4 egg whites
3 tablespoons zero-calorie sweetener suited for cooking and baking, such as Splenda

1. Line the inside of a soufflé dish with a strip of aluminum foil that should extend at least 1¼ inches above the top of the dish.
2. Place the yogurt in a medium bowl. Sift the cocoa powder through a fine sieve over the yogurt, then beat with an electric hand mixer until the yogurt and the cocoa powder are thoroughly combined.
3. In a mixing bowl, beat the egg whites with the sweetener until stiff.
4. Gently fold the egg whites into the cocoa mixture.
5. Pour the mixture into the prepared soufflé dish. The mixture should come up as far as the top of the dish.

6. Cover and place in the freezer for at least 3 hours.

7. When the soufflé is ready to eat, before serving, remove the aluminum foil and slice. Serve immediately.

Note: Raw or undercooked eggs should not be consumed by the very young, the very old, pregnant women, or anyone with a compromised immune system.

Oat Bran Cinnamon Chocolate Cookie

MAKES 1 SERVING

Preparation time: 5 minutes

Cooking time: 1 minute

2 tablespoons oat bran, such as Dukan Diet Organic Oat Bran

1 teaspoon low-fat cocoa powder, such as Dukan Diet Organic Cocoa Powder

⅛ teaspoon cinnamon

2 tablespoons fat-free milk

¼ teaspoon stevia, such as Dukan Diet Organic Stevia

1 drop almond extract

1. Mix all ingredients in a small bowl

2. Transfer cookie mix onto a microwave-safe plate and form into a cookie shape.

3. Microwave for 1 minute on high. For a crispier cookie, microwave on high for an additional minute and let cool for 2 minutes.

Dukan Nutella

MAKES 1 SERVING
Preparation time: 5 minutes
Cooking time: No cooking required

1 egg yolk
1 teaspoon low-fat cocoa powder, such as Dukan Diet Organic
Cocoa Powder
1 tablespoon zero-calorie sweetener suited for cooking and
baking, such as Splenda
1 drop almond extract

In a small bowl, whisk together the egg yolk, cocoa powder, sweetener, almond extract, and ¼ teaspoon water until smooth.

Note: Raw or undercooked eggs should not be consumed by the very young, the very old, pregnant women, or anyone with a compromised immune system.

Discover Dukan Diet Organic Cocoa Powder

Discover Dukan Diet Organic Oat Bran

Discover Dukan Diet Organic Stevia

──────── *Sauces and Dressings* ────────

Vinaigrette Maya

MAKES 2 SERVINGS
Preparation time: 35 minutes
Cooking time: No cooking required

1 tablespoon Dijon or French whole-grain mustard
5 tablespoons balsamic vinegar
1 teaspoon vegetable oil
1 garlic clove (optional)
7 to 8 fresh basil leaves, chopped
Salt and freshly ground black pepper

1. In a small bowl, combine the mustard, balsamic vinegar, vegetable oil, garlic (if using), and basil, plus salt and pepper to taste. Mix together until well blended.
2. Set aside for 30 minutes to infuse the garlic. Remove the garlic before serving.

Vinaigrette Bouillon

MAKES 2 SERVINGS
Preparation time: 10 minutes
Cooking time: No cooking required

1 low-sodium vegetable bouillon cube
1 level teaspoon cornstarch
2 tablespoons vinegar
1 tablespoon Dijon mustard or French whole-grain mustard

1. In a small bowl, combine the bouillon cube with 2 tablespoons of hot water. Stir until the cube dissolves.
2. Add the cornstarch, vinegar, and mustard, and whisk thoroughly.

Dukan Mayonnaise

MAKES 2 SERVINGS
Preparation time: 10 minutes
Cooking time: No cooking required

1 egg yolk
1 tablespoon Dijon mustard
Salt and freshly ground black pepper
1 tablespoon chopped fresh parsley or fresh chives
3 tablespoons fat-free plain Greek-style yogurt or fat-free
    ricotta (see Note)

1. In a small mixing bowl, combine the egg yolk and the mustard.
2. Season with salt and pepper to taste, and add the parsley or chives.
3. Gradually mix in the yogurt or ricotta, stirring continuously.
4. Refrigerate immediately.

Warning! Because of its raw egg content, mayonnaise must be kept chilled. This mayonnaise will keep refrigerated in a covered container for 2 to 3 days.
Note: If using ricotta, first process in a food processer until smooth.
Note: Raw or undercooked eggs should not be consumed by the very young, the very old, pregnant women, or anyone with a compromised immune system.

Dukan Mayonnaise II

MAKES 2 SERVINGS
Preparation time: 10 minutes
Cooking time: 20 minutes

1 egg
¼ cup fat-free plain Greek-style yogurt or fat-free ricotta
(see Note)
½ teaspoon Dijon mustard
Salt and freshly ground black pepper
½ teaspoon chopped fresh herbs, singly or mixed, such as
parsley, chives, or thyme (optional)

1. Place the egg in a large pot and cover with cold water.
2. Bring the water to a boil. Once the water is boiling, reduce to a simmer and cook the egg for 10 minutes.
3. Remove the egg from the hot water and help it cool by running cold water over it. Remove the shell, place the egg in a small bowl, and mash it with a fork.
4. Add the yogurt or ricotta to the mashed egg. Add the mustard, salt and pepper to taste, and herbs (if using). Combine thoroughly.
5. Refrigerate immediately.

Note: If using ricotta, first process in a food processer until smooth.

Ravigote Sauce

MAKES 4 SERVINGS
Preparation time: 10 minutes
Cooking time: 20 minutes

1 egg
3 medium sour, half-sour, or gherkin pickles, finely diced*
1 small onion, chopped
2 tablespoons chopped fresh chives
2 tablespoons chopped fresh parsley
2 tablespoons chopped fresh tarragon
1¼ cups fat-free plain Greek-style yogurt
½ teaspoon Dijon mustard
Salt

1. Place the egg in a large pot and cover with cold water. Bring the water to a boil. Once the water is boiling, reduce the heat to a simmer and cook the egg for 10 minutes.
2. Remove the egg from the hot water and help it cool by running cold water over it. Remove the shell and mash the egg in a small glass bowl.
3. Add the pickles, onion, chives, parsley, and tarragon.
4. Add the yogurt and mustard, plus salt to taste, and stir until thoroughly combined.

*Use only no-sugar-added pickles.

Note: Serve with fish, hard-boiled eggs, meat, or vegetables.

Onion Sauce

MAKES 4 SERVINGS
Preparation time: 10 minutes
Cooking time: 2 minutes

1 large onion, very finely chopped
½ cup low-sodium vegetable stock
1 egg yolk
2 tablespoons fat-free plain Greek-style yogurt
2 tablespoons fat-free ricotta
1 tablespoon vinegar
1 teaspoon mustard
Salt and freshly ground black pepper

1. In a saucepan, combine the onion and stock and bring to a boil over medium heat.
2. Reduce the heat to a simmer and cook for 2 minutes. Remove from the heat and let the mixture cool.
3. In a medium bowl, mix together the egg yolk, yogurt, ricotta, vinegar, and mustard, plus salt and pepper to taste.
4. Once the stock has cooled down, gradually add it to the egg yolk mixture, stirring thoroughly.

Note: Raw or undercooked eggs should not be consumed by the very young, the very old, pregnant women, or anyone with a compromised immune system.

Shallot Sauce

MAKES 6 SERVINGS
Preparation time: 10 minutes
Cooking time: 10 minutes

12 shallots, chopped
½ cup cider vinegar
¼ cup plus 1 teaspoon fat-free milk
1 egg yolk, beaten
Salt and freshly ground black pepper

1. Place the shallots in a saucepan with the vinegar and boil for 10 minutes.
2. Remove the mixture from the heat and add the milk and egg yolk. Stir vigorously, and season with salt and pepper to taste.

Yogurt and Fennel Sauce

MAKES 2 SERVINGS
Preparation time: 10 minutes
Cooking time: No cooking required

½ cup fat-free plain Greek-style yogurt
Juice of ½ lemon
Salt and freshly ground black pepper
2 small onions, chopped as fine as possible
½ fennel bulb, very finely chopped
1 teaspoon chopped fresh basil or fresh parsley

1. In a small bowl, combine the yogurt and the lemon juice. Season with salt and pepper to taste.
2. Add the onion, fennel, and basil and combine thoroughly.
3. Store in the refrigerator until ready to serve.

Spicy Red Pepper Sauce

MAKES 2 SERVINGS

Preparation time: 15 minutes, plus 1 hour for marinating

Cooking time: No cooking required

1 red bell pepper, stems and seeds removed, deseeded, and cut
  into very thin slices
1 garlic clove, chopped
½ onion, chopped
1 small fresh red chili, finely chopped
Juice of 1 lemon
Salt and freshly ground black pepper
⅛ teaspoon Tabasco sauce

1. In a small bowl, combine the red bell pepper, garlic, onion, chili pepper, and lemon juice. Season with salt and pepper to taste, and add Tabasco.
2. Allow the sauce to rest for at least 1 hour before serving.

Saffron Sauce

MAKES 2 SERVINGS

Preparation time: 2 minutes

Cooking time: No cooking required

1 teaspoon cornstarch
2 tablespoons low-sodium fish stock, at room temperature
A few saffron threads
Salt and freshly ground black pepper

1. In a small bowl, combine the cornstarch and fish stock. Mix until the cornstarch is dissolved.
2. Add the saffron and season with salt and pepper to taste.

Caper Sauce

MAKES 5 SERVINGS
Preparation time: 10 minutes
Cooking time: 15 minutes

2 tablespoons tomato purée
¼ cup fat-free milk
7 medium sour, half-sour, or gherkin pickles, chopped*
12 capers, drained and rinsed
Salt and freshly ground black pepper to taste

1. In a small saucepan, mix together the tomato purée and milk.
2. Add 2 tablespoons cold water and the pickles. Bring to a boil over medium heat, then reduce to a simmer and cook for 15 minutes.
3. Add the capers, and season with salt and pepper to taste.

*Use only no-sugar-added pickles.

Spinach Sauce

MAKES 4 SERVINGS
Preparation time: 10 minutes
Cooking time: 5 minutes

Salt
4 ounces spinach, washed
2 tablespoons fat-free plain Greek-style yogurt
½ cup low-sodium chicken stock
A pinch of grated nutmeg

1. Fill a pot with water, add a large pinch of salt, and bring to a boil. Add the spinach and blanch for 1 minute.
2. Drain the spinach, squeeze out the extra water, and blend it in a food processor or chop fine. Place in a medium bowl.

3. Add the yogurt, then gradually stir in the chicken stock.
4. Place the mixture in a saucepan and cook for 1 minute over high heat.
5. Season with nutmeg, and add salt to taste.

Herb Sauce

MAKES 2 SERVINGS
Preparation time: 15 minutes
Cooking time: 2 minutes

2 teaspoons cornstarch
2 garlic cloves, finely chopped
2 shallots, finely chopped
2 tablespoons fat-free plain Greek-style yogurt
3 sprigs of fresh parsley, finely chopped
3 sprigs of fresh tarragon, finely chopped
4 chives, finely chopped
Salt and freshly ground black pepper

1. In a small saucepan, combine the cornstarch with 1 tablespoon water.
2. Add the garlic, shallots, and yogurt.
3. Heat over low heat for 2 minutes, stirring continuously.
4. Add the parsley, tarragon, and chives. Season with salt and pepper to taste.

White Sauce

MAKES 3 SERVINGS
Preparation time: 5 minutes
Cooking time: 5 minutes

1 cup low-sodium chicken stock, chilled
2 tablespoons fat-free milk
1 tablespoon cornstarch
Salt and freshly ground black pepper
A pinch of ground nutmeg

1. In a small saucepan, mix together the chicken stock and milk. Gradually blend the cornstarch into the liquid.
2. Warm the mixture over low heat, stirring continuously with a wooden spoon, until it starts to thicken, about 5 minutes.
3. Remove the mixture from the heat, season with salt and pepper to taste, and add the nutmeg.

Chinese Mustard Sauce

MAKES 2 SERVINGS
Preparation time: 10 minutes
Cooking time: No cooking required

1 teaspoon wine vinegar
1 teaspoon mustard
1 pinch of ground ginger
Juice of 1 lemon
1 onion, very finely chopped
Salt and freshly ground black pepper

1. In a small bowl, mix together the vinegar, mustard, and ground ginger.
2. Add the lemon juice and onion, stirring continuously. Season with salt and pepper to taste.

Lemon and Chive Sauce

MAKES 4 SERVINGS
Preparation time: 10 minutes
Cooking time: No cooking required

Juice of ½ lemon
¾ cup fat-free plain Greek-style yogurt
1 bunch of fresh chives, finely chopped
Salt and freshly ground black pepper

1. In a small bowl, combine the lemon juice and yogurt.
2. Add the chives, and season with salt and pepper to taste.

Curry Sauce

MAKES 4 SERVINGS
Preparation time: 10 minutes
Cooking time: 20 minutes

1 egg
½ onion, finely chopped
1 teaspoon curry powder
¾ cup fat-free plain Greek-style yogurt

1. Place the egg in a large pot and cover with cold water. Bring the water to a boil. Once the water is boiling, reduce the heat to a simmer and cook the egg for 10 minutes.
2. Remove the egg from the hot water and help it cool by running cold water over it. Remove the shell, and separate the egg, placing the yolk in a small bowl and discarding the white.
3. In the small bowl, mash the egg yolk with a fork and mix in the onion and curry powder.
4. Gradually mix in the yogurt, stirring continuously.

Paprika and Red Pepper Sauce

MAKES 8 SERVINGS

Preparation time: 15 minutes

Cooking time: 1 hour

1 red bell pepper

1 yellow bell pepper

4 tomatoes

1 onion, chopped

1 teaspoon zero-calorie sweetener suited for cooking and
   baking, such as Splenda

3 tablespoons wine vinegar

A pinch of paprika

Salt and freshly ground black pepper

1. Turn the oven on to Broil.
2. Place the whole bell peppers on a baking sheet. Place the tray in the oven and cook, turning to cook on all sides, until charred, about 10 to 15 minutes.
3. Immediately place the peppers in a bowl and cover with a plate to steam.
4. Once the peppers have cooled, peel off the skin, cut in half, and remove the stems and seeds.
5. Fill a medium pot with water and bring to a boil. Add the tomatoes to the pot and poach for 30 seconds. Remove the tomatoes from the pot, peel off the skin, and remove the seeds.
6. In a blender, process the peppers, tomatoes, onion, sweetener, vinegar, and paprika until smooth, about 1 minute. Season with salt and pepper to taste,
7. Strain the puréed mixture into a saucepan.
8. Cover and cook over low heat for 40 minutes.

Grelette Sauce

MAKES 6 SERVINGS
Preparation time: 10 minutes
Cooking time: 5 minutes

4 tomatoes
½ cup fat-free plain Greek-style yogurt
5 shallots, chopped
Juice of 1 lemon
Salt and freshly ground black pepper

1. Fill a medium pot with water and bring to a boil. Add the tomatoes to the pot and poach for 30 seconds. Remove the tomatoes from the pot, drain, and peel off the skin.
2. In a blender, process the tomatoes, yogurt, shallots, and lemon juice until smooth, about 1 minute. Season with salt and pepper to taste.
3. Cover and refrigerate until served.

Lyonnaise Sauce

MAKES 3 SERVINGS
Preparation time: 10 minutes
Cooking time: No cooking required

½ cup fat-free plain Greek-style yogurt
1 tablespoon wine vinegar
Salt and freshly ground black pepper
1 garlic clove, very finely chopped
1 shallot, very finely chopped

1. In a small bowl, combine the yogurt and vinegar, and season with salt and pepper to taste.
2. Add the garlic and shallots, and whisk until thoroughly combined.

Gribiche Sauce

MAKES 8 SERVINGS

Preparation time: 10 minutes

Cooking time: 20 minutes

2 eggs

1 teaspoon mustard

1 tablespoon cider vinegar

Salt and freshly ground black pepper

1 teaspoon vegetable oil

1 cup fat-free plain Greek-style yogurt

1 shallot, chopped

3 medium sour, half-sour, or gherkin pickles, finely diced*

3 sprigs of fresh tarragon

1. Place the eggs in a large pot and cover with cold water.
2. Bring the water to a boil. Once the water is boiling, reduce the heat to a simmer and cook the eggs for 10 minutes.
3. Remove the eggs from the pot and help them to cool by running cold water over them.
4. Remove the shells and chop finely.
5. In a medium bowl, combine the mustard and vinegar, plus salt and pepper to taste. Whisk while slowly adding the oil until the sauce has emulsified.
6. Gradually add the yogurt, combining thoroughly.
7. Add the chopped hard-boiled eggs, shallot, pickles, and tarragon.
8. Season with salt and pepper to taste.

*Use only no-sugar-added pickles.

Béchamel Sauce

MAKES 6 SERVINGS

Preparation time: 10 minutes

Cooking time: 10 minutes

1 cup cold fat-free milk

1 tablespoon cornstarch

1 low-sodium beef bouillon cube

Salt and freshly ground black pepper

A pinch of ground nutmeg

1. In a small saucepan, mix together the milk and cornstarch and add the bouillon cube.
2. Cook for a few minutes over low heat until thick, stirring continuously.
3. Season with salt and pepper to taste, and add the nutmeg.

Hollandaise Sauce

MAKES 2 SERVINGS

Preparation time: 15 minutes

Cooking time: 5 minutes

1 egg, separated

1 teaspoon mustard

1 tablespoon fat-free milk

1 teaspoon lemon juice

Salt and freshly ground black pepper

1. In a medium heatproof bowl, combine the egg yolk, mustard, and milk.
2. Partially fill a medium pot with water and bring to a simmer.
3. Place the bowl with the egg yolk mixture over the pot. The bottom of the bowl should not touch the water.
4. Cook, whisking continuously, until the sauce thickens, taking care not to let it boil.

5. Remove the sauce from the heat and continue to whisk it while adding the lemon juice.

6. In a small mixing bowl, beat the egg white until stiff.

7. Carefully fold the egg white into the sauce. Season with salt and pepper to taste.

Note: Raw or undercooked eggs should not be consumed by the very young, the very old, pregnant women, or anyone with a compromised immune system.

Mustard Sauce

MAKES 6 SERVINGS
Preparation time: 10 minutes
Cooking time: 25 minutes

1 egg
2 teaspoons cornstarch
2 teaspoons vinegar, plus more if needed
2 teaspoons mustard
1 teaspoon chopped fresh herbs, singly or mixed, such as
     tarragon, chives, and thyme
Salt and freshly ground black pepper

1. Place the egg in a large pot and cover with cold water. Bring to a boil. Once the water is boiling, reduce the heat to a simmer and cook the egg for 10 minutes.

2. Remove the egg from the pot and help it cool by running cold water over it.

3. Remove the shell and separate the egg, placing the yolk in a small bowl and discarding the white.

4. In a medium bowl, combine the cornstarch with 1 tablespoon of cold water.

5. Place 1 cup of water in a small saucepan, bring to a boil, and whisk in the cornstarch mixture.

6. Reduce the heat, and simmer the cornstarch mixture for 3 minutes. Remove the mixture from the heat and cool.

7. In a food processor, process the egg yolk, vinegar, and mustard until smooth.
8. In a medium bowl, combine the egg yolk and the cornstarch mixtures.
9. Add the herbs, and season with salt and pepper to taste.
10. If the sauce is too thick, add more vinegar, ⅛ teaspoon at a time, until the desired consistency is reached.

Portuguese Sauce

MAKES 6 SERVINGS

Preparation time: 10 minutes

Cooking time: 30 minutes

8 tomatoes, stems and seeds removed, chopped
6 garlic cloves, crushed
2 medium onions, very finely chopped
2 dried bay leaves
Herbes de Provence (a mix of dried marjoram, thyme, savory, basil, rosemary, sage, and fennel seeds)
Salt and freshly ground black pepper
1 tablespoon tomato purée
1 green bell pepper, seeds removed, cut into very thin strips
A pinch of chili powder (optional)

1. In a medium pot, place the tomatoes, garlic, onions, bay leaves, and a few pinches of herbes de Provence. Cook over medium heat for 10 minutes. Season with salt and pepper to taste.
2. Add the tomato purée, reduce the heat to a simmer, and cook for an additional 20 minutes.
3. Remove the bay leaves.
4. In a food processor, blend the purée with the bell pepper until smooth, about 1 minute.
5. Add the chili powder (if using), pulse to combine. Serve warm.

Index

ABOUT THE AUTHOR

DR. PIERRE DUKAN has been a medical doctor specializing in human nutrition since 1973. He is the author of many works on nutrition for the scientific community, as well as works for the general public. He writes regularly in the press and appears on television. Dr. Dukan chairs R.I.P.O.S.T.E., an international association of nutritionists.

The popularity of Dr. Dukan's method and works in countries as different in culture as Korea and Bulgaria show how he has become the most widely read French nutritionist in the world. In 2009, *The Dukan Method* was the best-selling book in Poland.

Nowadays many health professionals and epidemiologists believe the Dukan Diet to be the method best equipped to put a halt to the weight problems that are still on the increase the world over.

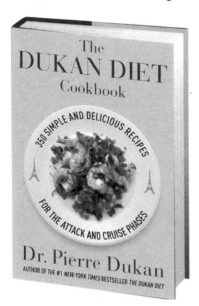
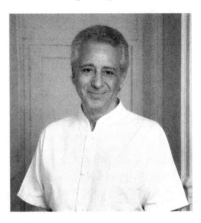
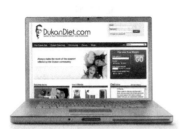
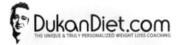
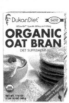

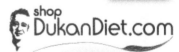